I0084332

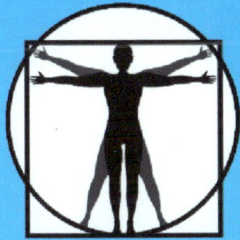

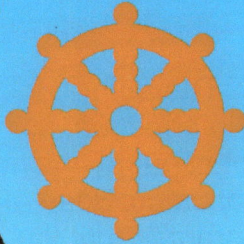

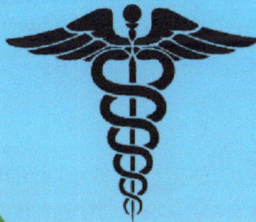

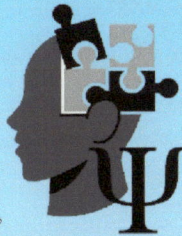

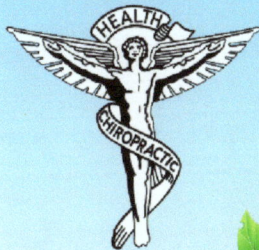

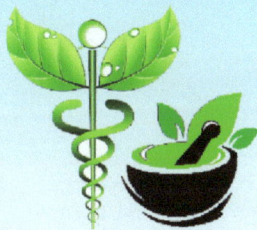

The Wellness Chronicles

Book 32

Volume 4

By Jim Moltzan

Insights on Holistic Health, Wellness, and Ancient Wisdom

Physical & Mental Well-being:
- Functional Anatomy
- Holistic Physiology
- Philosophy & Self-reflection
- Mind-Body Psychology
- Movement, Breath & Awareness

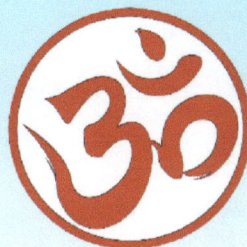

Disclaimer

This book is intended for information purposes only. The author does not promise or imply any results to those using this information, nor are they responsible for any adverse results brought about by the usage of the information contained herein. Use the information provided at your own risk. Furthermore, the author does not guarantee that the holder of this information will improve his or her health from the information contained herein.

The author of this book has used his/her best efforts in preparing this book. The author makes no representation of warranties with respect to the accuracy, applicability, or completeness of the contents of this book.

This book is © copyrighted by CAD Graphics, Inc. No part of this may be copied, or changed in any form, sold, or used in any way other than what is outlined within this book under any circumstances. No part of this book may be reproduced or transferred in any form or by any means, graphic, electronic, or mechanical, including photocopying, recording, taping, or by any information storage retrieval system, without the written permission of the author.

© 2025 CAD Graphics, Inc.

ISBN: 978-1-958837-42-9

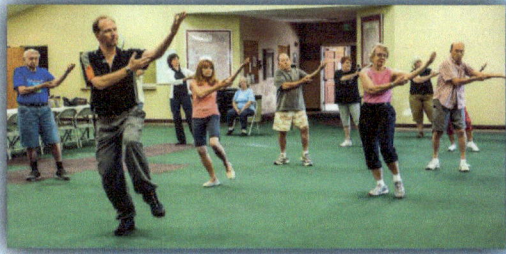

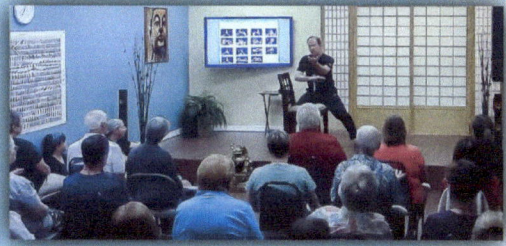

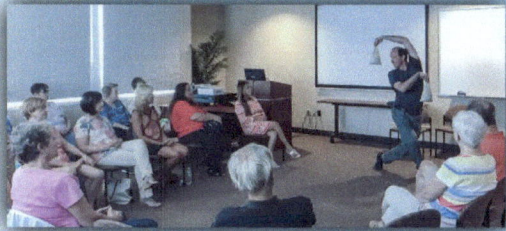

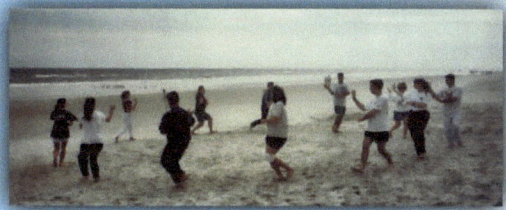

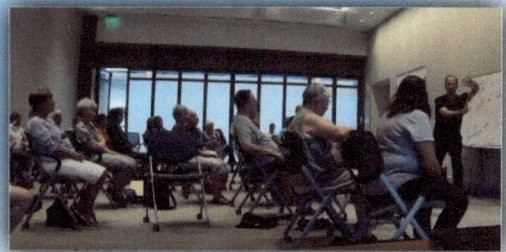

Foreword

I am honored to present *The Wellness Chronicles: Volume 4,* a further evolution of the ideas, reflections, and research I've cultivated over decades of personal practice and holistic exploration. This volume continues the path laid out in previous editions, drawing from hundreds of original writings, lectures, and graphics that span the intersection of body, mind, and spirit.

In our fast-paced, pharmaceutically dependent world, self-awareness and preventative health have become increasingly vital. This book offers not just knowledge, but a practical framework for reclaiming sovereignty over one's health and vitality. Within these pages, readers will find topics that span physiology, emotional resilience, the nervous system, breathing, posture, psychology, nutrition, and the often-overlooked spiritual dimension of well-being.

What sets this volume apart is its unapologetic confrontation with modern health crises of iatrogenic injuries, systemic medical failings, media distortion, and groupthink, all examined through a balanced lens of critical thinking and self-empowerment. At the same time, it honors timeless teachings from Traditional Chinese Medicine, Taoism, martial arts, Ayurveda, and contemplative philosophy, showing how these ancient systems offer practical guidance for contemporary challenges.

I have included many of my original graphics and illustrations to help convey these concepts visually, from the pathways of breath and energy to the structures of emotional and physical training. These visuals reinforce one of the book's central insights: that vitality arises from intentional balance between wind (breath), water (circulation), and fire (focus), echoing the Taoist concept that "wind and water create fire."

This is not a typical wellness book. It is a call to responsibility, to wisdom, to reflection and most of all, to action. Whether you're a seasoned practitioner or simply curious about taking control of your well-being, I invite you to walk this path with me. Learn, question, explore and integrate what resonates.

With sincerity and purpose,

Jim Moltzan

Why I Share, What I Have Learned

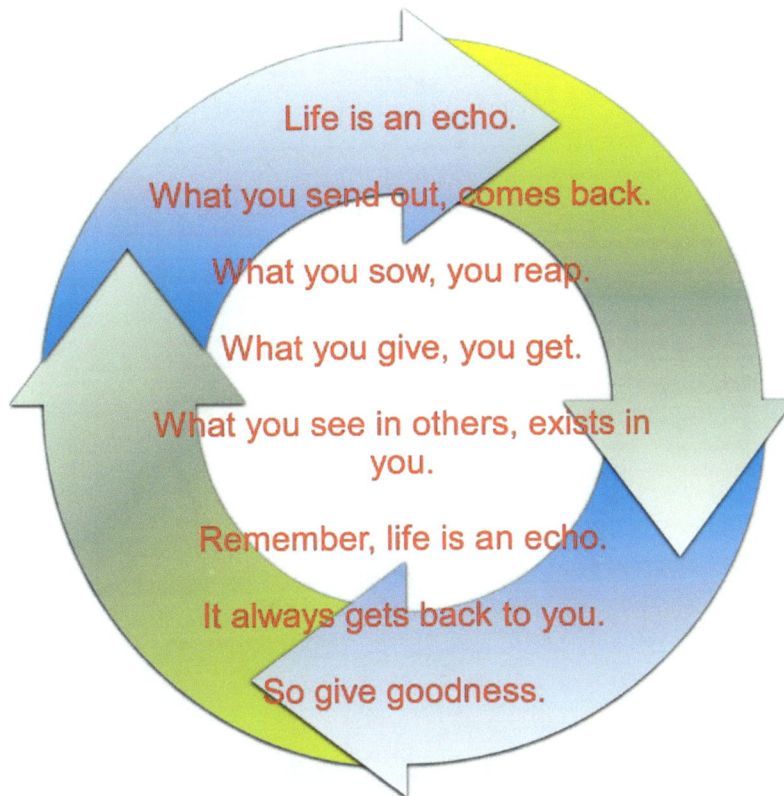

Life is an echo.

What you send out, comes back.

What you sow, you reap.

What you give, you get.

What you see in others, exists in you.

Remember, life is an echo.

It always gets back to you.

So give goodness.

www.MindAndBodyExercises.com

I made my commitment many years ago to learn, study, practice and teach fitness and well-being. My education came from martial arts and various other Eastern methods rooted in Traditional Chinese Medicine (TCM). I started when I was 16 years old and have never stopped since; 61 now.

I have written journals, produced educational graphics and co-authored a book in addition to many that I have self-authored. I blog often with a WordPress site, writing about the anatomical, physiological and mental benefits of mind and body training. Years back I started recording my classes and lectures, knowing that somewhere down the line, all of this information would be valuable to those who need and desire it.

My YouTube channel has almost 300 videos of FREE classes and other education videos. The goal all along has been to raise the awareness that Tai chi (a martial art), qigong (yoga at its root) and many other Eastern wellness methods, have proven the test of time for maintaining well-being. No gym, no mat, no membership, no special clothes or equipment. Just the individual and their engagement.

Weak or injured knees, back issues (strains & sciatica), stress & anxiety, asthma, arthritis, balance, poor posture - the list is endless. These are all issues that can be improved or overcome by those serious about learning about the mind, body & spirit connection.

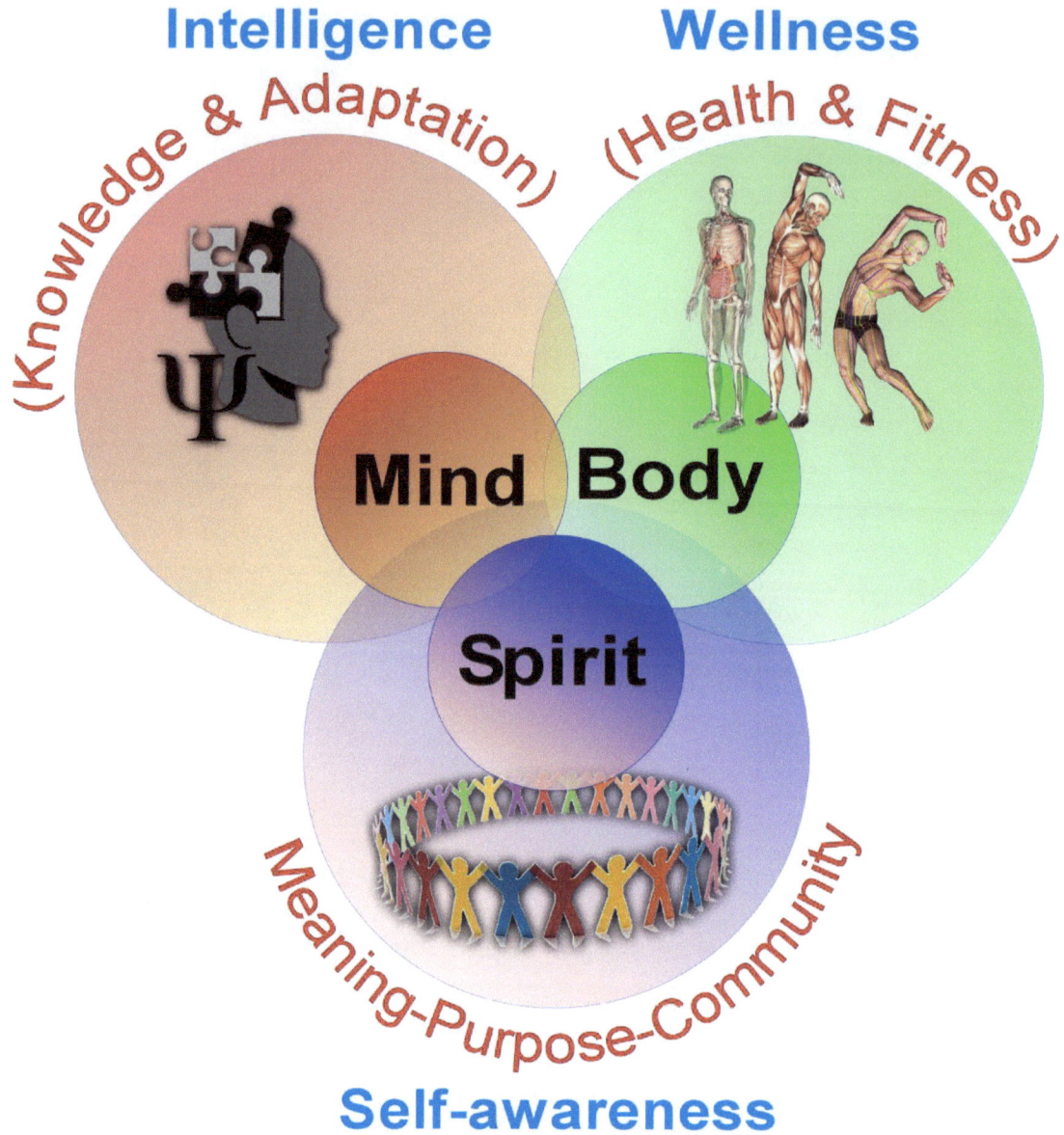

Intelligence   Wellness

(Knowledge & Adaptation)   (Health & Fitness)

Mind   Body

Spirit

Meaning-Purpose-Community

Self-awareness

We are the architect of our own health, happiness, destiny, or fate.

Table of Contents

SECTION I: Challenges in Modern Health Systems

Public health discussions often concentrate on contagious diseases such as measles, especially in light of recent outbreaks. In early 2025, the passing of a 6-year-old girl in Seminole, Texas, represented the first measles-related death in the United States in a decade (Bartlett, 2025). This event rekindled debates concerning vaccination and disease prevention strategies. Nonetheless, the significant focus on measles, despite its relatively low mortality rate, starkly contrasts with the limited dialogue surrounding iatrogenic injuries, which result in a substantial number of fatalities each year.

The Scope of the Issue: Measles vs. Iatrogenic Injuries

Measles: A Preventable Yet Overemphasized Disease
Measles, a highly contagious viral disease, was declared eliminated in the U.S. in 2000 but has resurfaced in communities with low vaccination rates. The recent Texas case highlighted the risks associated with vaccine hesitancy (Bartlett, 2025). Allopathic medical professionals consider measles preventable through the MMR (Measles, Mumps, and Rubella) vaccine, which is reported as 97% effective with two doses (CDC, 2025). However, concerns over vaccine safety and accountability persist. In 1986, Congress and President Reagan enacted the National Childhood Vaccine Injury Act (NCVIA), which created a system for compensating individuals harmed by vaccines while granting pharmaceutical companies' immunity from lawsuits related to vaccine injuries. This legislation has led to debates about vaccine mandates, corporate accountability, and public trust in immunization programs. Many feel that if the vaccines are safe and effective, why should a multi-billion-dollar industry not be held accountable for their products?

Iatrogenic Injuries: A Silent Epidemic

Iatrogenic injuries encompass medical errors, medication complications, surgical mistakes, and hospital-acquired infections. Research indicates that preventable medical errors contribute to over 400,000 deaths annually in the U.S., making them **the third largest leading cause of death in the US** (James, 2013). A widely cited study estimated approximately 250,000 iatrogenic deaths per year (Makary & Daniel, 2016). Dr. Barbara Starfield (2000) documented how **225,000** Americans die annually due to medical errors, including:

- **12,000** from unnecessary surgery
- **7,000** from medication errors in hospitals
- **20,000** from other hospital errors
- **80,000** from hospital-acquired infections
- **106,000** from adverse drug effects when taken as prescribed (Starfield, 2000).

Deadly Medical Errors in the US

Preventable medical mistakes are the third leading cause of death in the U.S. following heart disease and cancer.

250,000+
deaths every year in the U.S. from medical errors

Most Common Types of Cases

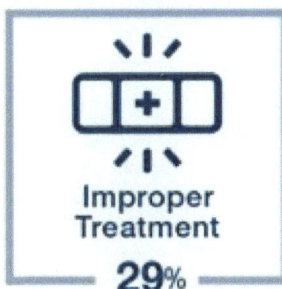

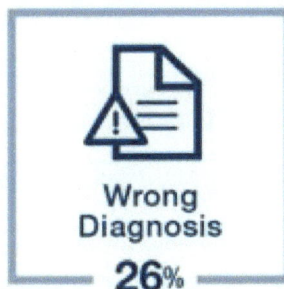

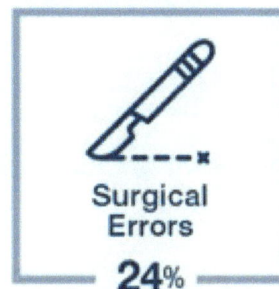

Improper Treatment	Wrong Diagnosis	Surgical Errors
29%	26%	24%

The remaining types of cases are obstetrics (5.4%), medication errors (5.1%), improper monitoring (3.8%), anesthesia errors (2.5%), and other (3.1%).

SOURCE: JOHN HOPKINS MEDICINE, JUSTPOINT

Death in the United States

Johns Hopkins University researchers estimate that medical error is now the third leading cause of death. Here's a ranking by yearly

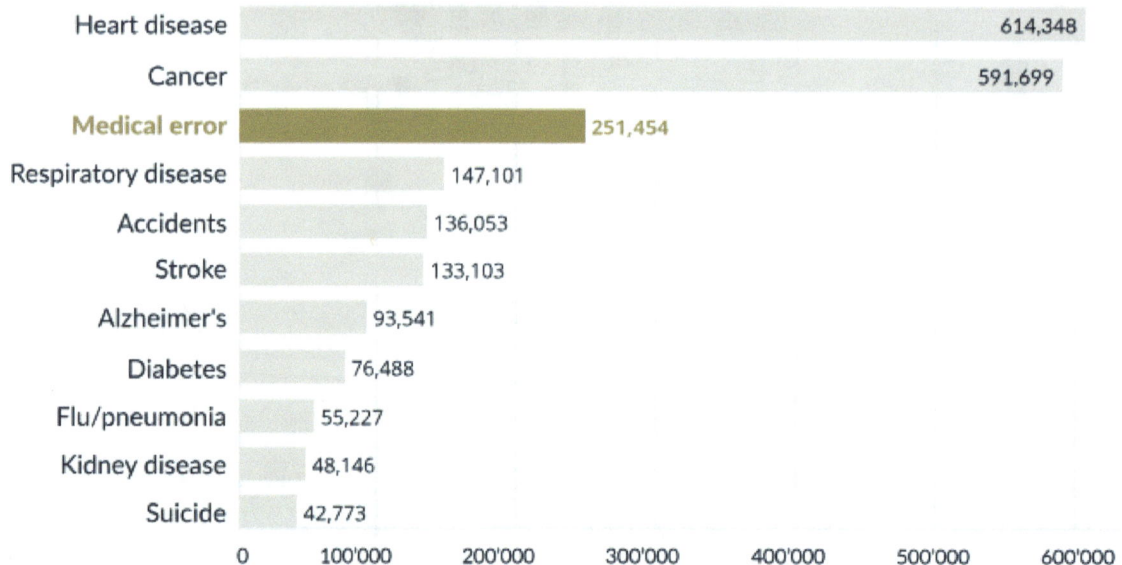

Cause	Deaths
Heart disease	614,348
Cancer	591,699
Medical error	**251,454**
Respiratory disease	147,101
Accidents	136,053
Stroke	133,103
Alzheimer's	93,541
Diabetes	76,488
Flu/pneumonia	55,227
Kidney disease	48,146
Suicide	42,773

Source:
https://www.washingtonpost.com/news/to-your-health/wp/2016/05/03/researchers-medical-errors-now-third-leading-cause-of-death-in-united-states/

Despite these alarming figures, public awareness and policy efforts remain disproportionately low compared to diseases like measles.

Why the Disparity in Media and Political Attention?

1. Media Sensationalism and Public Perception

Media outlets prioritize stories that generate fear and engagement. Measles outbreaks with their visible symptoms and high contagion make for dramatic headlines, while iatrogenic injuries occur behind hospital doors, lacking visual appeal for mass media (Bartlett, 2025).

2. Political and Public Health Priorities

Governments focus on highly contagious diseases like measles because they can cause widespread outbreaks. Vaccination campaigns offer a clear solution (WHO, 2024), whereas fixing medical errors needs systemic healthcare reforms, which are less appealing politically.

3. Institutional Interests and Liability

Acknowledging the extent of iatrogenic injuries necessitates systemic accountability from hospitals, pharmaceutical companies, and regulatory agencies, potentially resulting in legal implications and diminished public trust. Conversely, messaging regarding measles often supports pharmaceutical and public health objectives by promoting vaccination initiatives (WHO, 2024).

4. Public vs. Private Accountability

Measles outbreaks are often presented as a matter of public responsibility, with an emphasis on vaccine compliance. Conversely, iatrogenic injuries tend to be regarded as individual incidents rather than indicative of systemic issues, thus enabling healthcare institutions to evade thorough scrutiny (James, 2013).

5. Psychological Bias and Fear Appeal

Individuals tend to exhibit greater fear towards external, unpredictable threats, such as infectious diseases, compared to systemic risks, including medical errors. When measles is presented as an imminent crisis, it triggers a heightened fear response. In contrast, despite their significant impact, medical errors are frequently understated (Slovic, 2000).

The Need for a Balanced Approach

While any death is unfortunate, addressing measles outbreaks is vital. However, the focus on these outbreaks compared to iatrogenic injuries highlights an imbalance in public health priorities. Increasing transparency, implementing patient safety protocols, and facilitating discussions about medical errors are essential to reduce deaths and restore confidence in the US healthcare system.

The significant number of fatalities resulting from iatrogenic injuries highlights the critical need for enhanced patient safety protocols. A robust healthcare strategy must encompass both external health threats and internal systemic deficiencies to ensure better protection of patients' lives.

References:

Bartlett, T. (2025, March 11). *His daughter was America's first measles death in a decade*. The Atlantic. https://www.theatlantic.com/health/archive/2025/03/texas-measles-outbreak-death-family/681985/

Centers for Disease Control and Prevention (CDC). (2025, March 7). *Measles cases and outbreaks*. https://www.cdc.gov/measles/data-research/index.html

James, J. T. (2013). A new, evidence-based estimate of patient harms associated with hospital care. *Journal of Patient Safety, 9*(3), 122-128. https://doi.org/10.1097/PTS.0b013e3182948a69

Makary, M. A., & Daniel, M. (2016). Medical error—the third leading cause of death in the US. *BMJ, 353*, i2139. https://doi.org/10.1136/bmj.i2139

Starfield, B. (2000). Is US health really the best in the world? *JAMA, 284*(4), 483-485. https://doi.org/10.1001/jama.284.4.483

Slovic, P. (2000). *The perception of risk*. Earthscan Publications.

World Health Organization (WHO). (2024, November 14). *Measles fact sheet*. https://www.who.int/news-room/fact-sheets/detail/measles

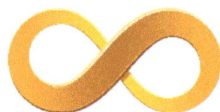

In contemporary society, the credibility of the healthcare system is frequently called into question. Despite significant investment in U.S. healthcare, exceeding $4 trillion annually, the system often prioritizes profit over prevention and wellness. This profit-driven approach, heavily influenced by pharmaceutical companies, insurance corporations, and healthcare systems, has resulted in patients being viewed as long-term customers rather than individuals empowered to manage their own health. Although emergency and acute care services in the U.S. are commendable, there is a concerning trend regarding the prevention of chronic diseases and the maintenance of long-term well-being (Hurley et al., 2024).

The Healthiest (& Unhealthiest) Countries in the World

Health and health care system index scores by country (100=best possible score)

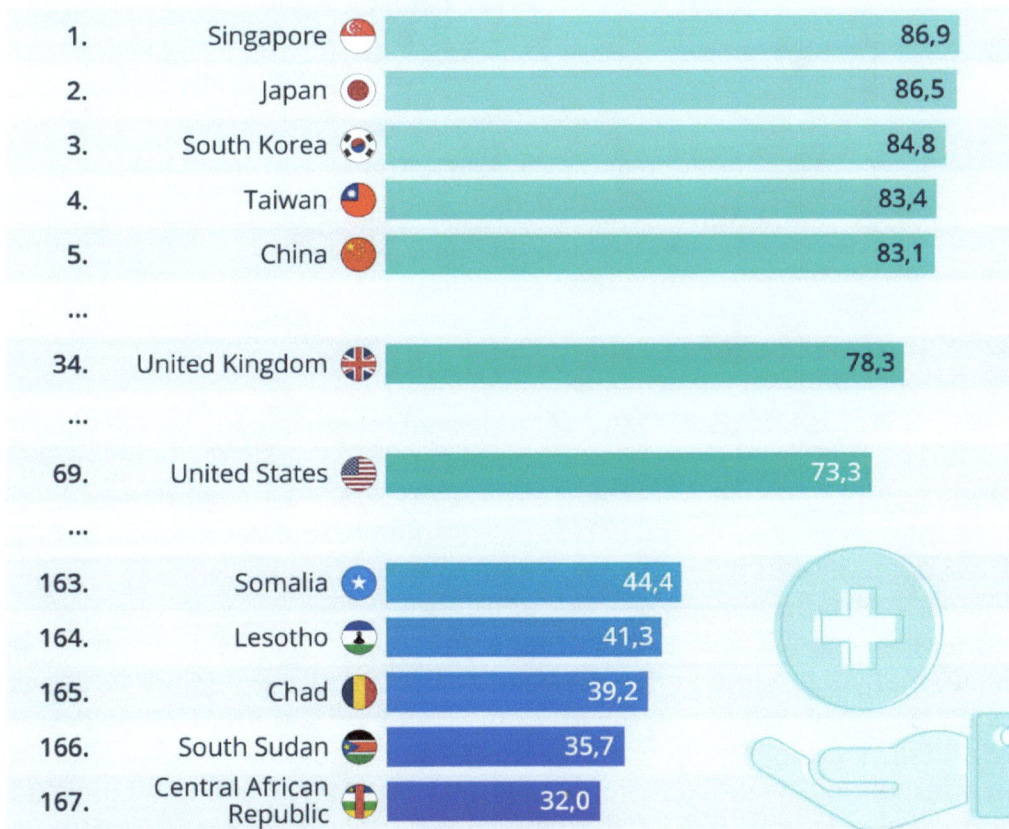

1.	Singapore	86,9
2.	Japan	86,5
3.	South Korea	84,8
4.	Taiwan	83,4
5.	China	83,1
...		
34.	United Kingdom	78,3
...		
69.	United States	73,3
...		
163.	Somalia	44,4
164.	Lesotho	41,3
165.	Chad	39,2
166.	South Sudan	35,7
167.	Central African Republic	32,0

* Based on people's health, access to health services, health outcomes, health systems, illness and risk factors, mortality rates. 2022 or latest available

Source: Legatum Institute Foundation

statista

The Role of Trust in Healthcare

Skepticism regarding healthcare is understandable when one examines the statistics. For instance, the U.S. experiences a concerning 250,000 to 400,000 iatrogenic deaths annually, those resulting from medical intervention (Makary & Daniel, 2016). However, this represents only one perspective. The other perspective highlights that despite significant healthcare expenditure, the system performs poorly in terms of life expectancy and chronic disease management compared to other affluent nations (Health at a Glance 2019, 2019). Numerous factors contribute to this issue, including an over-reliance on medications and surgeries, which frequently result in complications rather than the prevention of diseases (Sackett, 2000).

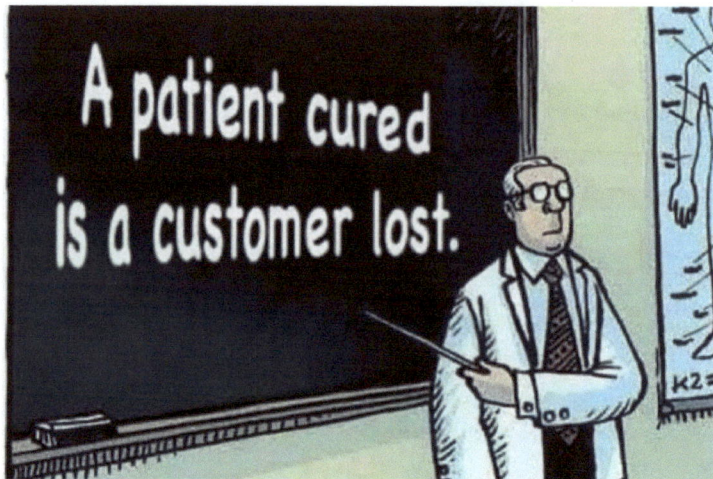

Medical Dissent and the Cost of Speaking Out

Historically, medical professionals who question prevailing narratives have frequently encountered scrutiny, censorship, and professional consequences. Recently, numerous highly esteemed doctors and scientists have expressed concerns regarding public health policies, vaccine mandates, and the influence of pharmaceutical companies, only to face discreditation or suppression.

While healthcare professionals with solid credentials have raised concerns about the current state of medicine, many have encountered backlash. Distinguished doctors such as Dr. Daniel Neides have questioned the safety and efficacy of certain medical interventions (Dyer, 2017), and Dr. Peter McCullough despite being one of the most published cardiologists in the world, had his medical board certifications challenged due to him expressing his concerns regarding the medical industry's response to the COVID-19 pandemic (Hulscher et al., 2023). Despite their efforts to initiate important discussions, these professionals often experience a loss of credibility among the public and their peers, being labeled as outliers or conspiracy theorists (Hoffman et al., 2021).

Dr. Robert Malone, a scientist important in developing mRNA vaccine technology, has raised concerns about the safety and long-term effects of these vaccines. Despite his contributions,

8

Malone was deplatformed from major social media platforms after questioning the COVID-19 vaccine rollout and advocating for caution (*In-Depth: Did Robert Malone Invent mRNA Vaccines in San Diego?* 2022). His case highlights the issue of scientists facing professional ostracization when their views diverge from mainstream policies.

Dr. Mary Talley Bowden, a specialist in ear, nose, and throat medicine, became involved in controversy due to her public support for alternative early treatments and her criticism of vaccine mandates. Consequently, she was suspended from Houston Methodist Hospital. Undeterred, she established her own independent practice, where she continues to treat patients based on her medical observations and research (Bowden, 2022). Her experience highlights the increasing divide between institutional medicine and the physicians who advocate for personalized care.

Dr. Alex Cole, a medical researcher and clinician, has expressed concerns about the transparency of vaccine safety data. He has emphasized the importance of open scientific debate and the inclusion of alternative viewpoints. The key issue is whether medical professionals should experience professional consequences for participating in legitimate scientific discussions (Professional, 2024).

Other doctors, including Dr. Pierre Kory, a critical care specialist, and Dr. Paul Marik, an intensive care expert, have discussed the perceived limitations of the mainstream approach to COVID-19 treatments. They have supported the use of repurposed drugs and alternative treatment protocols, which resulted in professional examination and debate. Dr. Kory and Dr. Marik encountered resistance when promoting these alternative COVID-19 treatment strategies (Marik et al., 2020).

These cases highlight a trend in modern medicine where differing opinions, even those from individuals with significant experience and expertise, are often dismissed rather than discussed. Scientific progress relies on thorough discussion and analysis, yet the current environment frequently favors conformity over inquiry. Regardless of individual perspectives on these particular matters, the marginalization of seasoned professionals poses ethical and scientific questions about transparency, accountability, and the impact of influential industries on medical dialogue.

The Case for Personal Responsibility in Health

With the system seemingly failing at times, many individuals are choosing to take responsibility for their own health. Rejecting the mainstream "sick care" model, which often prioritizes a "pill for every ill," people are turning to alternative practices that emphasize prevention, self-care, and holistic wellness. Taking responsibility for one's own health through practices like tai chi, qigong, (VA Office of Patient Centered Care and Transformation, n.d.), martial arts, yoga, meditation and even weight training have become powerful ways for individuals to manage stress, improve physical fitness, and maintain mental clarity.

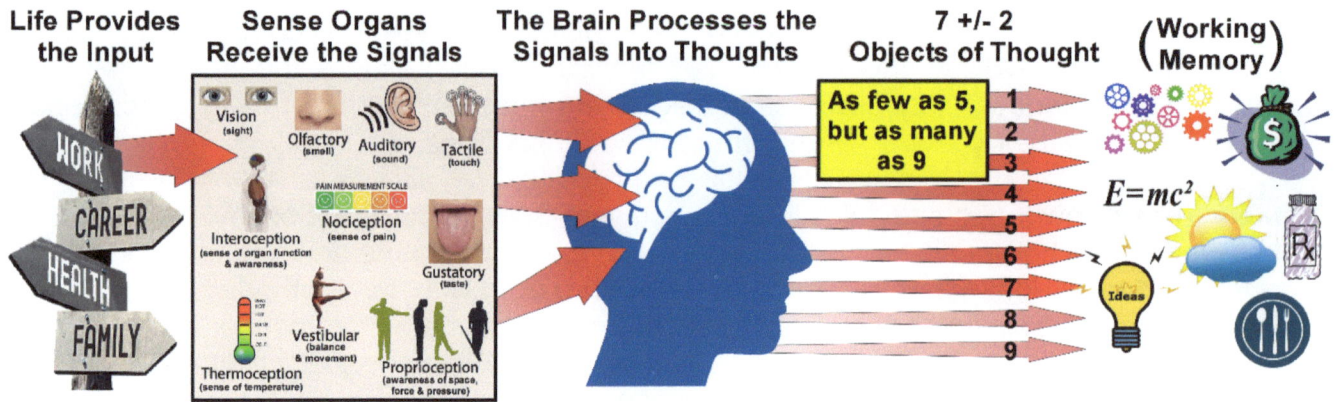

Life Provides the Input	Sense Organs Receive the Signals	The Brain Processes the Signals Into Thoughts	7 +/- 2 Objects of Thought	(Working Memory)

For me, personally, the approach is clear: read labels, carefully monitor what goes in, on, and around the body, practice daily exercises to strengthen the body, and employ stress management techniques for the mind and soul. I limit my mental intake by reducing exposure to the news and social media, focusing instead on the bigger picture. While I cannot change the world, I know I can change myself and influence those around me in a positive way.

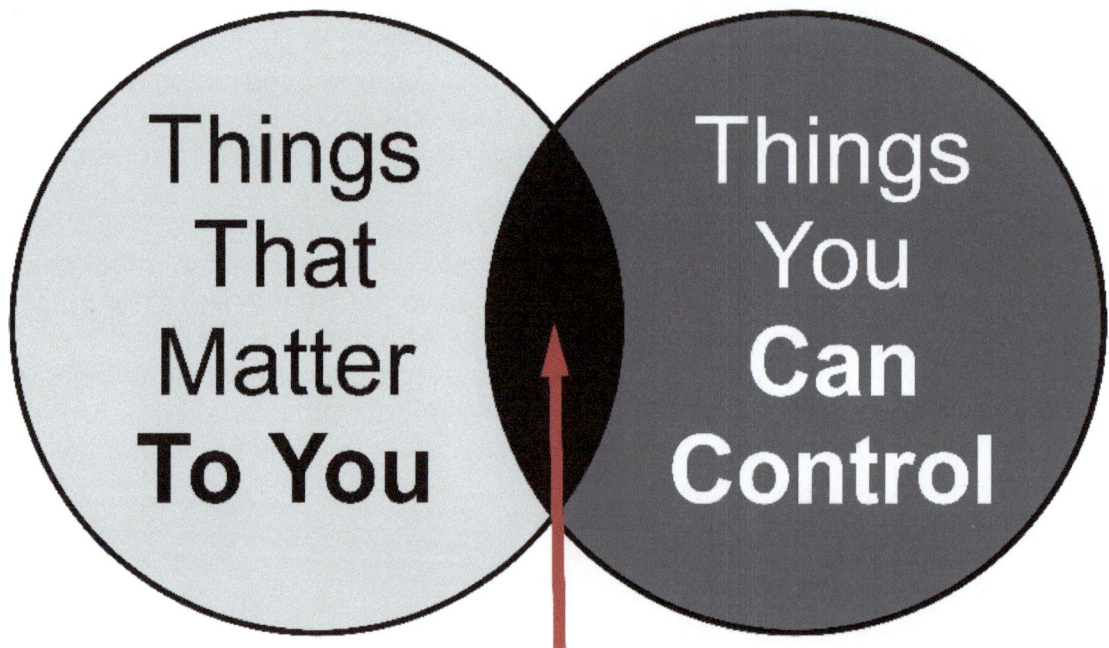

Things That Matter To You

Things You Can Control

What You Should Put Energy Towards

The Need for Change

Moving toward a preventative and holistic healthcare approach is crucial, despite challenges in a profit-driven system. The influence of pharmaceutical companies, insurance, and large healthcare interests often overlooks patient well-being (Dickinson, 2014). A shift to a system that rewards prevention, empowers individuals, and values overall well-being over chronic condition management is needed.

However, comprehensive change may be challenging to achieve at the national level. At the individual level, however, transformation is feasible. By taking personal responsibility for our health instead of solely relying on a system that may prioritize profit over care, we make an empowering choice. Engaging in alternative and preventive practices, such as tai chi, qigong, yoga, resistance training or daily meditation, enables us to regain control over our wellness incrementally.

References:

Bowden, M. T. (2022, March 6). *Fighting Methodist Hospital — BREATHEMD | Optimal Airway Health*. BREATHEmd | Optimal Airway Health. https://breathemd.org/blog/2022/2/27/the-story-behind-why-im-suing-the-hospital-who-suspended-me-for-prescribing-ivermectin

Dickinson, J. (2014, April 1). *Deadly medicines and organised crime: How big pharma has corrupted healthcare*. https://pmc.ncbi.nlm.nih.gov/articles/PMC4046551/

Dyer, O. (2017). Cleveland Clinic to re-evaluate its Wellness Institute after director questions vaccines. *BMJ*, j253. https://doi.org/10.1136/bmj.j253

Health At a Glance 2019. (2019, November 7). OECD. https://www.oecd.org/en/publications/health-at-a-glance-2019_4dd50c09-en.html

Hoffman, D., Stewart, A., Breznay, J., Simpson, K., & Crane, J. (2021). Vaccine hesitancy narratives. *Voices in Bioethics*, 7. https://doi.org/10.52214/vib.v7i.8789

Hulscher, N., Procter, B. C., Wynn, C., & McCullough, P. A. (2023). Clinical Approach to Post-acute Sequelae After COVID-19 Infection and Vaccination. *Cureus*, *15*(11), e49204. https://doi.org/10.7759/cureus.49204

Hurley, B., Lovett, S., D'Urso, J., & Smith, E. (2024, December 14). Three medical bills that show true cost of America's 'broken' healthcare. *The Times*. https://www.thetimes.com/world/us-world/article/us-healthcare-insurance-companies-ceo-shooting-z597qlq2n?utm_source=chatgpt.com®ion=global

In-Depth: Did Robert Malone invent mRNA vaccines in San Diego? (2022, January 27). UC Irvine News. https://news.uci.edu/2022/01/27/in-depth-did-robert-malone-invent-mrna-vaccines-in-san-diego/

Makary, M. A., & Daniel, M. (2016). Medical error—the third leading cause of death in the U.S. *BMJ*, 353, i2139. https://doi.org/10.1136/bmj.i2139

Marik, P. E., Kory, P., Varon, J., Iglesias, J., & Meduri, G. U. (2020). MATH+ protocol for the treatment of SARS-CoV-2 infection: the scientific rationale. *Expert Review of Anti-infective Therapy*, *19*(2), 129–135. https://doi.org/10.1080/14787210.2020.1808462

Professional, C. C. M. (2024, December 4). *Informed consent*. Cleveland Clinic. https://my.clevelandclinic.org/health/articles/24268-informed-consent
Sacket, D. (2000) *Evidence-based medicine : how to practice and teach EBM : Free Download, Borrow, and Streaming : Internet Archive.* (2000). Internet Archive. https://archive.org/details/evidencebasedmed00davi/mode/2up?q=reliance

VA Office of Patient Centered Care and Transformation. (n.d.). TAI CHI AND QI GONG. In *VA Office of Patient Centered Care and Cultural Transformation* (pp. 1–7). https://www.va.gov/WHOLEHEALTHLIBRARY/docs/Tai-Chi-and-Qi-Gong.pdf

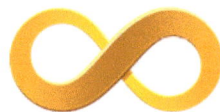

Throughout history, some products initially approved by regulatory agencies such as the U.S. Food and Drug Administration (FDA) and the Environmental Protection Agency (EPA) have later been found to pose risks to human health and the environment. While human error is sometimes unavoidable, minimizing it is crucial for public safety and welfare. From pharmaceuticals to household products, these instances underscore the importance of thorough testing and evaluation. This article examines notable cases such as thalidomide, DDT, and OxyContin, and discusses strategies to prevent similar issues in the future.

Thalidomide: The Drug That Never Reached the U.S. (Officially)

Thalidomide was introduced in the 1950s by the German company Chemie Grünenthal as a sedative and treatment for morning sickness in pregnant women. It was marketed in Europe, Canada, and other countries as a completely safe medication. However, by the late 1950s, a significant number of children were born with severe congenital disabilities, including missing or deformed limbs, organ damage, and other critical conditions (Kim & Scialli, 2011).

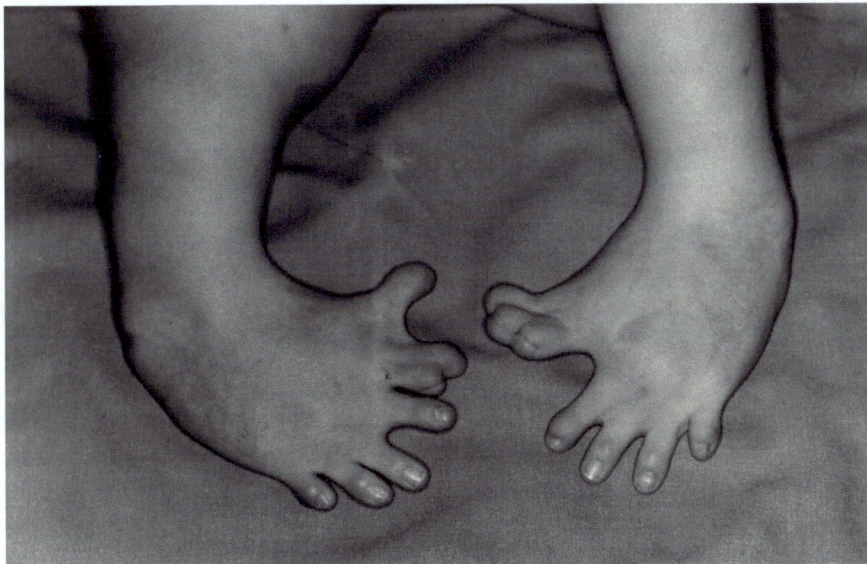

Why Wasn't Thalidomide Approved in the U.S.?

The pharmaceutical company submitted the drug for FDA approval, but Dr. Frances Kelsey, a physician and pharmacologist at the FDA, halted its approval. She requested additional safety data due to suspected potential hazards. As a result of her diligence, the United States avoided a significant public health disaster (Daemmrich, 2004).

Although not approved, certain U.S. doctors were able to access the drug through experimental trials. Approximately 17 children in the United States were born with birth defects associated with thalidomide (Kim & Scialli, 2011). While this figure is relatively small compared to the over 10,000 cases worldwide, it underscores the risks involved with unregulated drug distribution. Thalidomide resulted in significant modifications to drug approval processes globally, including enhanced testing for fetal safety and stricter FDA guidelines that continue today (Daemmrich, 2004).

DDT: The Miracle Pesticide Turned Environmental Nightmare

DDT (Dichlorodiphenyltrichloroethane) was introduced in the 1940s as a pesticide to address malaria and typhus. It was widely used by the U.S. military during World War II and subsequently gained popularity in agriculture and public health programs (Eskenazi et al., 2009).

By the 1960s, concerns about the environmental and health impacts of DDT became more prominent. Rachel Carson's seminal book, *Silent Spring* (1962), documented the bioaccumulation of DDT in wildlife, which resulted in the thinning of bird eggshells and contributed to the near-extinction of bald eagles. Additionally, Carson highlighted potential carcinogenic effects of DDT on humans (Carson, 1962).

DDT was prohibited in the United States in 1972; however, it continues to be utilized in certain regions globally for malaria control (Eskenazi et al., 2009).

OxyContin & the Opioid Epidemic: A Tragic Case of Corporate Deception

In 1996, Purdue Pharma launched OxyContin, promoting it as a non-addictive pain medication. The Food and Drug Administration (FDA) approved the drug based on Purdue's assertions that its time-release formulation would mitigate the potential for abuse (Van Zee, 2009).

OxyContin has been associated with high addiction rates, and its widespread prescription contributed to a national opioid crisis. Purdue Pharma and other manufacturers later faced lawsuits, with evidence suggesting that they did not fully disclose the drug's risks to doctors and regulators (Van Zee, 2009).

The opioid crisis has led to over **500,000 overdose deaths** in the United States since the late 1990s (*Uncovering the Opioid Epidemic*, n.d.). Although current opioid regulations are significantly stricter, the consequences of the crisis persist.

Vioxx: The Painkiller That Led to Heart Attacks

Vioxx (Rofecoxib), a medication for arthritis, was released in 1999 and marketed as an alternative to older anti-inflammatory drugs. Subsequent studies indicated that Vioxx was associated with an increased risk of heart attacks and strokes (Graham et al., 2005).

14

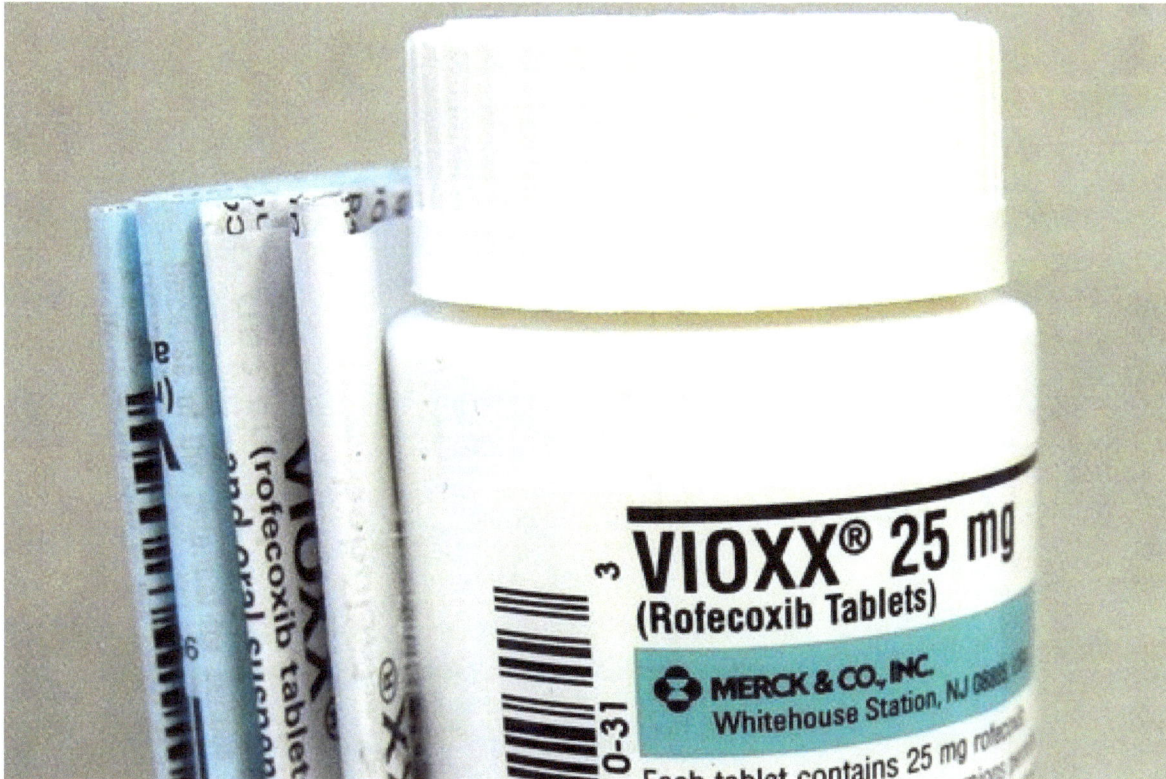

By the time Vioxx was withdrawn from the market, it is estimated that 20 million Americans had taken the drug. Research later published in the medical journal *Lancet* estimates that 88,000 Americans experienced heart attacks due to taking Vioxx, with 38,000 fatalities (Prakash, 2007). This case underscored the inadequacy of drug companies in disclosing safety risks and led to the implementation of more stringent post-market drug surveillance policies.

Other Notable Cases of "Safe" Products That Became Harmful:

◆ **Tobacco:** Once promoted as doctor-approved, later linked to lung cancer and heart disease (Centers for Disease Control and Prevention (US), 2014)

◆ **Lead Paint & Leaded Gasoline:** Used for decades despite known toxicity, leading to widespread **neurological damage** in children (Needleman, 2004).

◆ **Asbestos:** Used in construction for insulation, but later found to cause mesothelioma and lung disease (Bolan et al., 2023)

◆ **Baby Powder (Talc):** Contaminated with **asbestos**, leading to lawsuits over ovarian cancer risks (Cramer et al., 2015)

◆ **Frontal Lobotomies:** Once considered a treatment for mental illness, but resulted in severe cognitive impairment and even death (Faria, 2013)

◆ **Agent Orange:** A herbicide used during the Vietnam War, later linked to cancer and birth defects (Stellman & Stellman, 2018)

◆ **PFAS ("Forever Chemicals"):** Found in water supplies and linked to **cancer, infertility, and immune disorders** (Ayodele & Obeng-Gyasi, 2024)

Lessons Learned & How to Protect Ourselves Today:

Question Corporate Claims: Research beyond marketing as companies may prioritize profits over safety.

Demand Rigorous Testing: Ensure drugs and chemicals undergo long-term studies before use.

Advocate for Transparency: Pressure is crucial to release hidden data on harmful products.

Support Independent Research: Prioritize independent, peer-reviewed research over industry-funded studies.

Stay Informed: Be vigilant about new risks like microplastics in food and AI-driven medical decisions.

References:

Ayodele, A., & Obeng-Gyasi, E. (2024). Exploring the Potential Link between PFAS Exposure and Endometrial Cancer: A Review of Environmental and Sociodemographic Factors. *Cancers, 16*(5), 983. https://doi.org/10.3390/cancers16050983

Bolan, S., Kempton, L., McCarthy, T., Wijesekara, H., Piyathilake, U., Jasemizad, T., Padhye, L. P., Zhang, T., Rinklebe, J., Wang, H., Kirkham, M., Siddique, K. H., & Bolan, N. (2023). Sustainable management of hazardous asbestos-containing materials: Containment, stabilization and inertization. *The Science of the Total Environment, 881*, 163456. https://doi.org/10.1016/j.scitotenv.2023.163456

Carson, R. (1962). *Silent spring.* Houghton Mifflin.

Centers for Disease Control and Prevention (US). (2014). *The Health Consequences of Smoking—50 years of progress.* NCBI Bookshelf. https://www.ncbi.nlm.nih.gov/books/NBK179276/

Cramer, D. W., Vitonis, A. F., Terry, K. L., Welch, W. R., & Titus, L. J. (2015). The association between Talc use and ovarian cancer. *Epidemiology, 27*(3), 334–346. https://doi.org/10.1097/ede.0000000000000434

Daemmrich, A. (2004). *Pharmacopolitics: Drug regulation in the United States and Germany.* UNC Press Books.
Eskenazi, B., Chevrier, J., Rosas, L. G., Anderson, H. A., Bornman, R., Bouwman, H., ... & Warner, M. (2009). The Pine River statement: Human health consequences of DDT use. *Environmental Health Perspectives, 117*(9), 1359-1367.

Faria, M. (2013). Violence, mental illness, and the brain - A brief history of psychosurgery: Part 1 - From trephination to lobotomy. *Surgical Neurology International, 4*(1), 49. https://doi.org/10.4103/2152-7806.110146

File:NCP14053.jpg – Wikimedia Commons. (n.d.). https://commons.wikimedia.org/wiki/File:NCP14053.jpg

Graham, D. J., Campen, D., Hui, R., Spence, M., Cheetham, C., Levy, G., Shoor, S., & Ray, W. A. (2005). Risk of acute myocardial infarction and sudden cardiac death in patients treated with cyclo-oxygenase 2 selective and non-selective non-steroidal anti-inflammatory drugs: nested case-control study. *The Lancet, 365*(9458), 475–481. https://doi.org/10.1016/s0140-6736(05)17864-7

Kim, J. H., & Scialli, A. R. (2011). Thalidomide: The tragedy of birth defects and the effective treatment of disease. *Toxicological Sciences, 122*(1), 1-6.
Needleman, H. (2004). Lead poisoning. *Annual Review of Medicine, 55*(1), 209–222. https://doi.org/10.1146/annurev.med.55.091902.103653

Prakash, S. (2007, November 10). Timeline: The rise and fall of Vioxx. *NPR.* https://www.npr.org/2007/11/10/5470430/timeline-the-rise-and-fall-of-vioxx

Rockoff, J. (2009, November 24). Vioxx and heart attack linked in 2001. *WSJ.* https://www.wsj.com/articles/SB10001424052748704779704574554071807123380

Stellman, J. M., & Stellman, S. D. (2018). Agent Orange during the Vietnam War: the lingering issue of its civilian and military health impact. *American Journal of Public Health, 108*(6), 726–728. https://doi.org/10.2105/ajph.2018.304426

Van Zee, A. (2009). The promotion and marketing of OxyContin: Commercial triumph, public health tragedy. *American Journal of Public Health, 99*(2), 221-227. https://doi.org/10.2105/AJPH.2007.131714

Uncovering the opioid epidemic. (n.d.). https://www.cdc.gov/museum/pdf/cdcm-pha-stem-uncovering-the-opioid-epidemic-lesson.pdf

Why Some Doctors Risk Their Careers to Question Mainstream Medicine

Public trust in physicians and hospitals has decreased significantly since the COVID-19 pandemic, with a notable drop from 71.5% in April 2020 to 40.1% in January 2024. This decline in trust is associated with factors like age, gender, lower educational level, income, and rural living (Hibbert, 2024). However, In recent years, a growing number of doctors and medical professionals have taken bold and often controversial stances that challenge mainstream medical paradigms. These individuals, many of whom have established careers and financial stability, risk their reputations and livelihoods to question the safety and efficacy of widely accepted interventions, particularly vaccination. Their actions raise an important question: *Why would accomplished professionals jeopardize their careers when there is seemingly little to gain?* The answer lies in a convergence of ethical convictions, clinical observations, and growing concerns about the influence of industry on public health.

Moral and Ethical Convictions

For many dissenting doctors, the decision to speak out is rooted in their ethical obligation to protect patient well-being. The Hippocratic Oath, which emphasizes "doing no harm," compels these professionals to prioritize the safety of their patients, even when their views place them at odds with the medical establishment. Dr. Suzanne Humphries, a nephrologist and co-author of *Dissolving Illusions: Disease, Vaccines, and the Forgotten History*, is one such example. Humphries transitioned from conventional nephrology to integrative medicine after observing patterns in her patients that led her to question the safety and effectiveness of vaccines (Humphries & Bystrianyk, 2013). Her journey reflects a broader trend among doctors who feel morally compelled to share their findings despite the potential consequences.

Firsthand Experiences and Clinical Pattern Recognition

Many of these professionals cite their clinical experiences as the catalyst for their change in perspective. They report encountering unexpected adverse reactions, inconsistencies between patient outcomes and established guidelines, and patterns that contradict the mainstream narrative. When such observations accumulate, they often prompt these doctors to dig deeper into medical history, epidemiological data, and alternative research, leading them to challenge conventional wisdom. Humphries (2013) highlights that her shift in perspective began after observing kidney patients suffering from vaccine-related complications, which prompted her to investigate the history of vaccines and public health.

Disillusionment with the Medical System

A growing number of physicians have become disillusioned with the modern medical system, which they believe prioritizes pharmaceutical interventions over addressing the root causes of disease. These doctors argue that the system operates within a profit-driven framework that emphasizes symptom management rather than long-term health promotion. As medical protocols increasingly align with pharmaceutical interests, some professionals feel constrained by hospital policies and insurance limitations that discourage holistic or preventative approaches to care.

Scientific Integrity and the Spirit of Inquiry

Another motivating factor for these dissenting professionals is their commitment to scientific integrity and open inquiry. Science, by its very nature, thrives on questioning established paradigms and re-evaluating conclusions in light of new evidence. However, many of these doctors argue that the current medical landscape discourages open debate, often labeling dissenting voices as "misinformation" without addressing their concerns. Humphries and Bystrianyk (2013) emphasize the importance of revisiting historical data and re-examining the role of vaccines in disease decline, advocating for a more nuanced understanding of public health history.

Concerns About Censorship and Suppression

Many doctors who speak out also point to the growing suppression of alternative viewpoints in medicine and public health. They argue that meaningful scientific progress requires open dialogue and that silencing dissenting voices undermines public trust. When legitimate concerns about vaccine safety, adverse reactions, and long-term consequences are dismissed without consideration, these doctors feel compelled to advocate for a more balanced discussion.

Intrinsic Motivation and Legacy

For some, the decision to challenge mainstream medical practices stems from a profound sense of purpose and desire to make a lasting impact. After decades of practice, these professionals often feel they have little to lose but much to gain by advocating for what they believe is right. Their motivation extends beyond financial gain or career advancement, reflecting a genuine desire to protect public health and encourage informed decision-making.

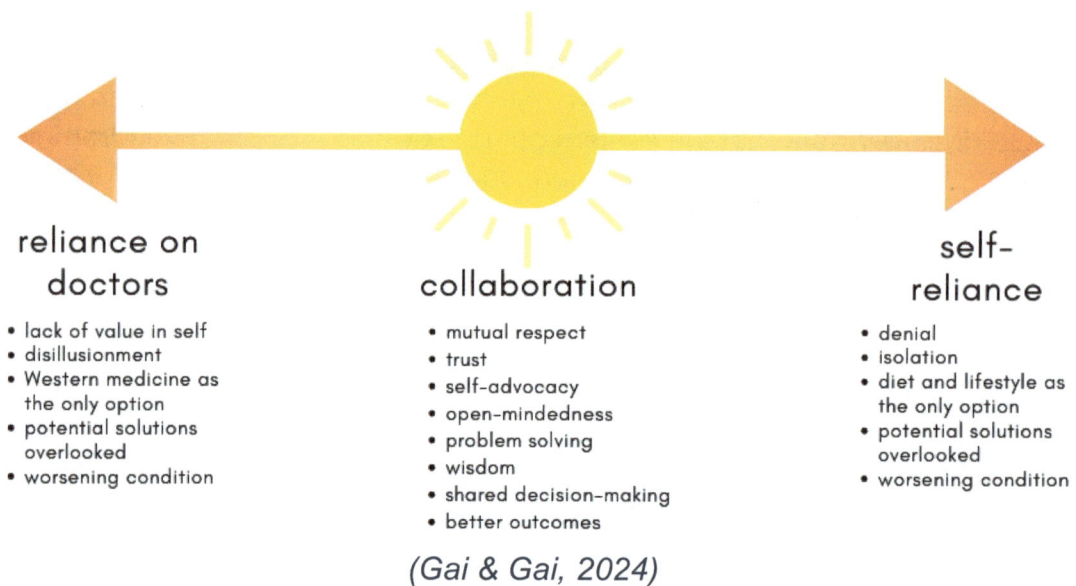

reliance on doctors
- lack of value in self
- disillusionment
- Western medicine as the only option
- potential solutions overlooked
- worsening condition

collaboration
- mutual respect
- trust
- self-advocacy
- open-mindedness
- problem solving
- wisdom
- shared decision-making
- better outcomes

self-reliance
- denial
- isolation
- diet and lifestyle as the only option
- potential solutions overlooked
- worsening condition

(Gai & Gai, 2024)

Are They on to Something?

Given the risks involved, it is worth considering whether these professionals might be highlighting genuine gaps and biases in the medical establishment. Their critiques often align with concerns about:

- Over-reliance on pharmaceutical interventions.

- Insufficient emphasis on lifestyle, nutrition, and preventive care.

- Long-term consequences of mass vaccination and immune system dysregulation.

- Lack of informed consent and transparency regarding potential risks.

While their views challenge mainstream paradigms, history has shown that dissenting voices have often been instrumental in driving scientific progress. Galileo's heliocentric theory and Semmelweis's (1861) advocacy for handwashing were once considered heretical but eventually transformed scientific understanding. Likewise, today's dissenting doctors may be raising critical questions that deserve serious consideration and further investigation.

Conclusion

The decision of respected doctors and medical professionals to challenge established medical norms is most often not driven by financial gain or career advancement. Rather, it is rooted in ethical convictions, clinical observations, and a commitment to scientific inquiry. As these voices grow louder, they encourage a much-needed conversation about the safety, efficacy, and long-term consequences of medical interventions. Their willingness to question prevailing narratives may ultimately lead to a more balanced, patient-centered approach to healthcare.

References:

Gai, & Gai. (2024, August 1). When you've lost trust in doctors. . . » Global Autoimmune Institute. *Global Autoimmune Institute »*. https://www.autoimmuneinstitute.org/articles/when-youve-lost-trust-in-doctors/

Hibbert, C. M. (2024, August 7). Trust in physicians and hospitals plummeted since the COVID pandemic, Northeastern research says. *Northeastern Global News*. https://news.northeastern.edu/2024/08/07/trust-in-physicians-hospitals-research/

Humphries, S., & Bystrianyk, R. (2013). *Dissolving illusions: Disease, vaccines, and the forgotten history*. CreateSpace Independent Publishing Platform.

Semmelweis, I. (1861). *Die Ätiologie, der Begriff und die Prophylaxis des Kindbettfiebers*. C.A. Hartleben's Verlags-Expedition.

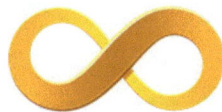

Rising Health Concerns Since 2020: A Holistic Overview of Emerging Trends

Since 2020, public attention has largely focused on infectious diseases such as COVID-19 and vaccine-preventable illnesses like measles and tuberculosis. However, an alarming rise in several chronic, developmental, and mental health conditions suggests a deeper crisis in population health, especially in the United States. This article outlines key health trends that deserve greater attention, including sudden cardiac events, mental health disorders, obesity and type 2 diabetes in adolescents, and the resurgence of various cancers.

Sudden Cardiac Death and Vascular Events

Sudden cardiac death (SCD), once relatively rare among young adults, has shown an increase in prevalence. Between 1999 and 2020, the age-adjusted mortality rate for SCD among U.S. adults aged 25-44 rose from 0.10 to 0.18 per 100,000; a significant public health concern (The Cardiology Advisor, 2025). Additionally, deaths from aortic aneurysms have become more frequent among adults, though definitive recent data is still emerging.

Infant Mortality and Early-Life Risk

The U.S. infant mortality rate rose by 3% in 2022 to 5.6 deaths per 1,000 live births, the first increase in two decades. The rise was especially significant in states like Georgia, Texas, and Missouri, and among infants born to White and Native American women. Contributing factors include maternal health complications and bacterial sepsis (Falconer, 2023).

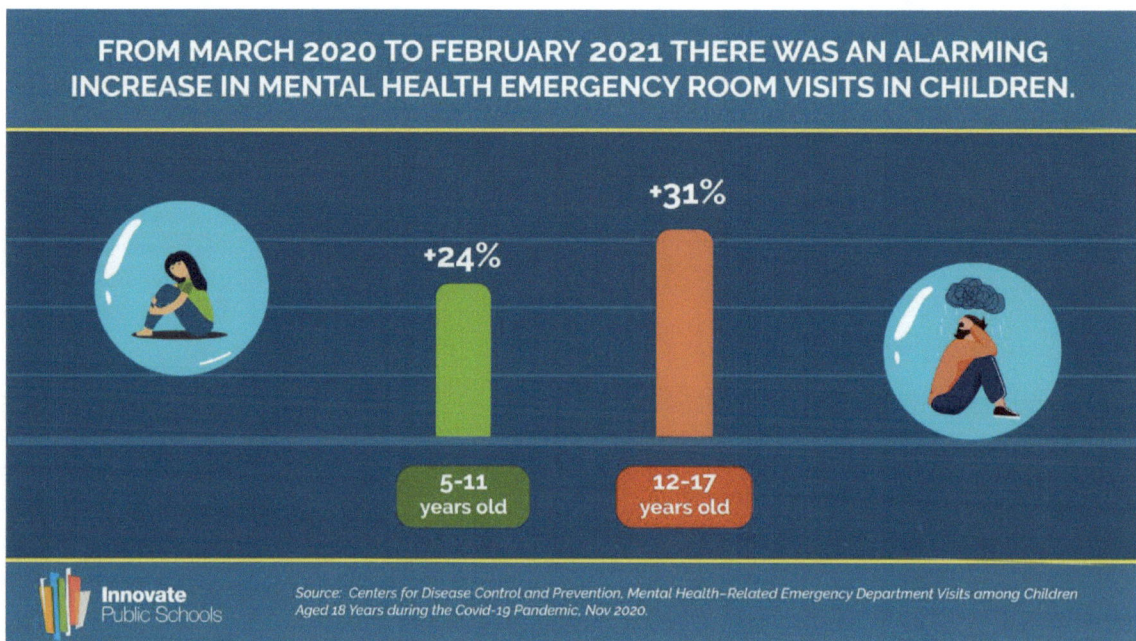

FROM MARCH 2020 TO FEBRUARY 2021 THERE WAS AN ALARMING INCREASE IN MENTAL HEALTH EMERGENCY ROOM VISITS IN CHILDREN.

+24% 5-11 years old
+31% 12-17 years old

Source: Centers for Disease Control and Prevention, Mental Health–Related Emergency Department Visits among Children Aged 18 Years during the Covid-19 Pandemic, Nov 2020.

Innovate Public Schools

(Winston & Winston, 2022)

Mental Health Crisis and Suicide

The COVID-19 pandemic has exacerbated mental health conditions, particularly among adolescents and young adults. Increased rates of anxiety, depression, and suicide have been documented, with long-term consequences expected. A significant contributing factor has been the reduction in school-based mental health support following the expiration of pandemic relief funding (Houston Chronicle, 2024).

Adolescent Obesity and Type 2 Diabetes

Obesity affects nearly 1 in 5 U.S. youth aged 2-19 years, with disproportionately high rates among Hispanic and non-Hispanic Black populations ((*Childhood Obesity Facts*, 2024). Concurrently, the incidence of type 2 diabetes in adolescents has risen sharply. Projections suggest a 700% increase by 2060 if current trends continue (*Diabetes in Young People Is on the Rise*, 2024).

Alzheimer's Disease: A Looming Epidemic

Currently, over 6.9 million Americans aged 65 and older are living with Alzheimer's disease. This figure is expected to double to 13.8 million by 2060 due to aging demographics and unknown environmental and lifestyle factors (Alzheimer's Association, 2024).

Colorectal and Pancreatic Cancers in Younger Adults

Although colorectal cancer rates have declined overall due to better screening in older adults, incidence in younger populations (ages 25-50) has doubled since 1995. Advanced-stage diagnoses are increasing at a rate of 3% annually in adults under 50 (American Cancer Society, 2023). Similarly, pancreatic cancer is on the rise, particularly among young women, with experts noting a significant and concerning shift in the disease burden (Harnisch-Weidauer, 2024).

Conclusion

The rise in both communicable and non-communicable diseases since 2020 signals a multi-faceted public health challenge. While infectious diseases tend to dominate media cycles, chronic conditions, mental health issues, and early-onset cancers are equally pressing. These trends underscore the urgent need for holistic prevention strategies, health education, and early interventions that go beyond vaccination campaigns and address root causes like nutrition, stress, environmental toxicity, and healthcare inequality.

References:

Alzheimer's Association. (2024). *2024 Alzheimer's disease facts and figures*.
https://pubmed.ncbi.nlm.nih.gov/38689398/
American Cancer Society. (2023). *Colorectal Cancer Facts & Figures 2023-2025*.
https://www.cancer.org/content/dam/cancer-org/research/cancer-facts-and-
statistics/colorectal-cancer-facts-and-figures/colorectal-cancer-facts-and-figures-2023.pdf

Childhood obesity Facts. (2024, April 2). Obesity. https://www.cdc.gov/obesity/childhood-
obesity-facts/childhood-obesity-facts.html

Diabetes in young people is on the rise. (2024, May 15). Diabetes.
https://www.cdc.gov/diabetes/data-research/research/young-people-diabetes-on-rise.html

Falconer, R. (2023, November 1). U.S. infant mortality rate rises for first time in over 2
decades. *Axios*. https://www.axios.com/2023/11/01/us-infant-mortality-rate-rises-first-time-
two-decades

Harnisch-Weidauer, L. (2024, November 18). *What you need to know about rising pancreatic
cancer rates*. Dana-Farber Cancer Institute. https://blog.dana-
farber.org/insight/2024/11/what-you-need-to-know-about-rising-pancreatic-cancer-rates/

Houston Chronicle. (2024). *Mental health crisis in students persists post-COVID*.
https://www.houstonchronicle.com/news/houston-texas/education/hisd/article/texas-covid-
mental-health-crisis-20205168.php

Partain, C. (2025, March 13). Houston students' mental health still hasn't rebounded from
COVID. *Houston Chronicle*. https://www.houstonchronicle.com/news/houston-
texas/education/hisd/article/texas-covid-mental-health-crisis-20205168.php

The Cardiology Advisor. (2025, March 5). *Sudden cardiac death rate increasing for younger
adults in the US*. https://www.thecardiologyadvisor.com/news/sudden-cardiac-death-rate-
increasing-for-younger-adults-in-the-us/

Winston, S., & Winston, S. (2022, May 13). *COVID-19 has harmed students' social-emotional
wellbeing, making it even more difficult to learn | Innovate Public Schools*. Innovate Public
Schools | a World-Class Public School for Every Student.
https://innovateschools.org/research-and-data/learning-loss/covid-19-has-harmed-students-
social-emotional-wellbeing-making-it-even-more-difficult-to-learn/

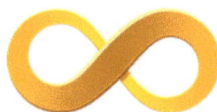

The Meat We Eat: Are We Consuming Chronic Illness?

Modern society is grappling with a chronic disease epidemic, with most Americans suffering from comorbidities and taking multiple pharmaceuticals daily. However, while we focus on human health, we often overlook a parallel crisis, one happening within the animals we consume. If humans are chronically ill, is it reasonable to assume that animals raised in industrial farming operations are immune? The reality is that livestock experience chronic illness due to poor diets, pharmaceutical overuse, and unnatural living conditions. As a result, humans ingest not only nutrients but also the byproducts of disease and drug residues.

1. Livestock and Chronic Illness: A Hidden Epidemic

Just as human health is compromised by poor nutrition and sedentary lifestyles, industrially raised livestock suffer from chronic illnesses caused by unnatural diets and overcrowding.

- **Antibiotic Overuse:** Animals in factory farms receive antibiotics to promote growth and prevent disease in unsanitary conditions. This practice fuels antibiotic-resistant bacteria, a serious threat to human health (Landers et al., 2012).

- **Chronic Inflammation:** Livestock fed grain-based diets (instead of grass) develop inflammation, fatty liver disease, and immune dysfunction, mirroring the harms of processed foods in humans (Apaoblaza et al., 2019).

- **Hormonal Imbalances:** Growth hormones and synthetic chemicals disrupt animals' endocrine systems, with potential effects on human consumers (Vandenberg et al., 2012).

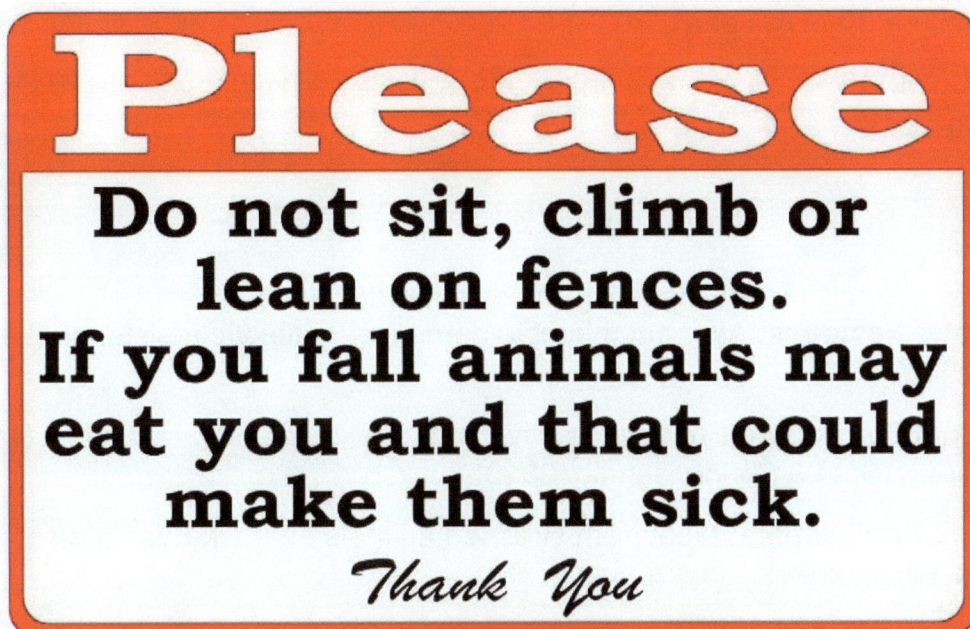

Please
Do not sit, climb or lean on fences.
If you fall animals may eat you and that could make them sick.
Thank You

2. Poor Nutrition, Poor Health: Consequences of Unnatural Diets

Processed foods have deteriorated human health, and similarly, commercial animal diets lack natural nutrition, fostering disease.
- **Cattle on Grain Diets:** Cows evolved to eat grass but are fed grains, causing acidosis, liver abscesses, and immune suppression (Russell & Rychlik, 2001).

- **Chickens and Confinement:** Factory-farmed chickens endure respiratory infections and skeletal deformities due to overcrowding (Mench et al., 2010).

- **Pigs and Stress-Related Illnesses:** Intelligent and stressed in confinement, pigs face weakened immunity and higher disease rates (Marchant-Forde, 2009).

3. Pharmaceutical Dependence: Treating Symptoms, Not Causes

Industrial farming mirrors healthcare's symptom-focused approach, relying on drugs to sustain unhealthy conditions.
- **Antibiotics and Vaccines:** Routine use prevents infections in filthy environments but breeds antibiotic-resistant bacteria (Laxminarayan et al., 2013).

- **Growth Hormones:** Recombinant bovine somatotropin (rBST) increases milk production but causes metabolic stress (Dohoo et al., 2018).

4. Genetic Manipulation: Creating Fragile Animals

Selective breeding for rapid growth yields biologically compromised animals.
- **Broiler Chickens:** Bred to grow unnaturally fast, they suffer musculoskeletal and organ failure (Knowles et al., 2008).

- **Dairy Cows:** High milk production breeds mastitis and metabolic disorders (Oltenacu & Broom, 2010).

5. The Impact on Human Health: You Are What Your Food Eats

Consuming sick animals means ingesting illness byproducts:
- **Antibiotic Residues:** Alter gut microbiota and fuel antibiotic resistance (Laxminarayan et al., 2013).

- **Hormonal Disruption:** Endocrine-active compounds in animal fat affect fertility and metabolism (Soto & Sonnenschein, 2010).

- **Inflammatory Profiles:** Meat from stressed animals exacerbates chronic inflammation (Most & Yates, 2021)

6. The Paradox of Industrial Farming: A Broken System

Like modern healthcare, industrial farming masks symptoms instead of solving root causes:

- **Symptom Management:** Drugs sustain sick animals in unnatural environments.

- **Profit Over Health:** High yields come at the cost of animal and human health.

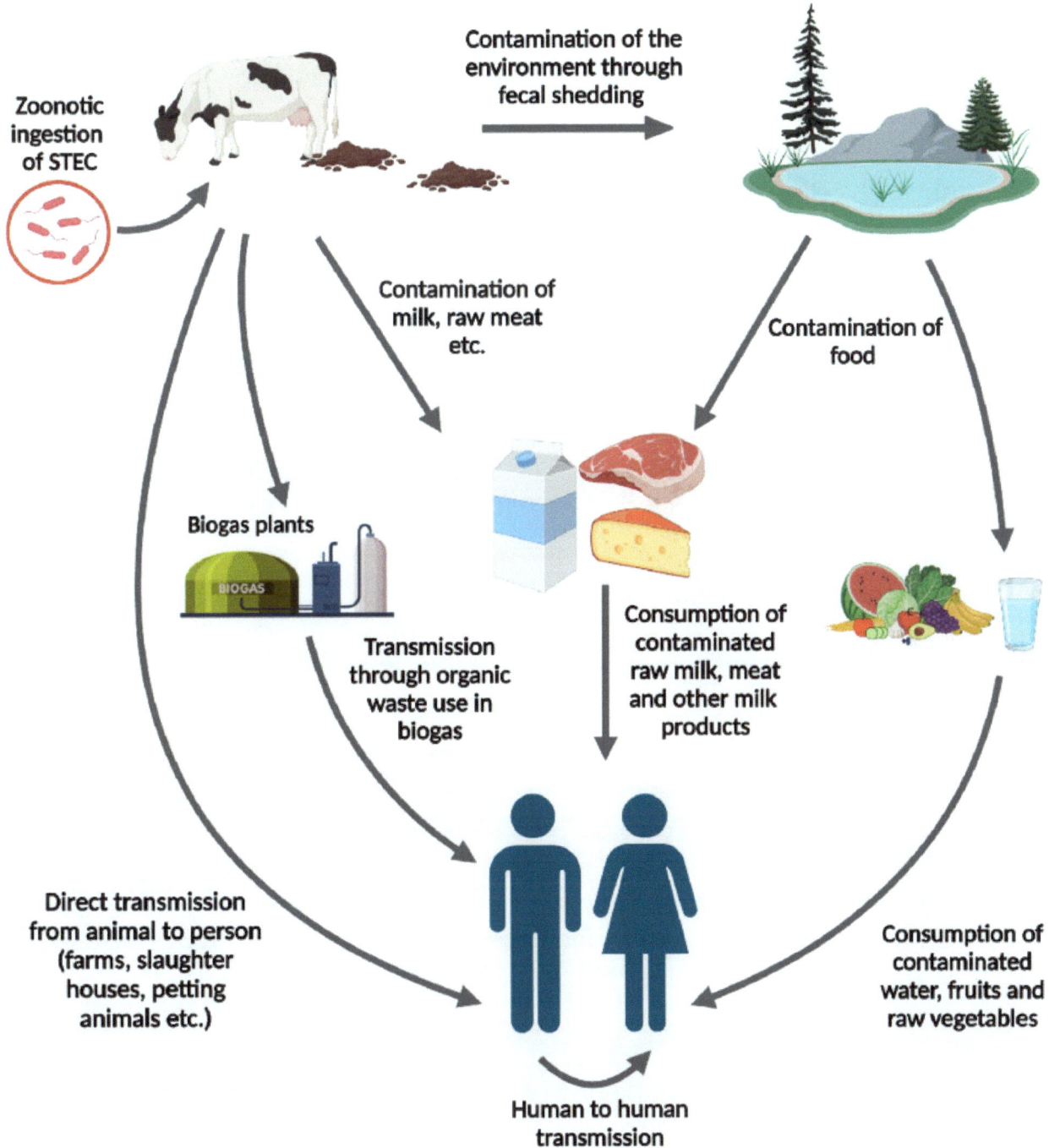

(Edison et al., 2024)

7. Solutions: Regenerative Agriculture and Conscious Consumption

Breaking the cycle is possible:

- **Pasture-Raised, Grass-Fed Meat:** Healthier and free from pharmaceuticals (Daley et al., 2010).

- **Organic and Local Farming:** Reduces chemical exposure and supports biodiversity (Reganold & Wachter, 2016).

- **Diversified Diets:** Plant-based proteins reduce reliance on factory-farmed meat.

Final Thoughts: The Ripple Effect of Conscious Choices

Choosing ethically raised meat improves human health and supports a system that prioritizes wellness for all beings. The health of animals and humans is inextricably linked—conscious choices can break the cycle of chronic illness.

References:

Daley, C. A., Abbott, A., Doyle, P. S., Nader, G. A., & Larson, S. (2010). A review of fatty acid profiles and antioxidant content in grass-fed and grain-fed beef. *Nutrition Journal, 9*(1), 10. https://doi.org/10.1186/1475-2891-9-10

Dohoo, I. R., Leslie, K., DesCôteaux, L., Fredeen, A., Dowling, P., Preston, A., & Shewfelt, W. (2003). A meta-analysis review of the effects of recombinant bovine somatotropin. 1. Methodology and effects on production. Canadian journal of veterinary research = Revue canadienne de recherche veterinaire, 67(4), 241–251.

Apaoblaza, A., Gerrard, S., Matarneh, S., Wicks, J., Kirkpatrick, L., England, E., Scheffler, T., Duckett, S., Shi, H., Silva, S., Grant, A., & Gerrard, D. (2019). Muscle from grass- and grain-fed cattle differs energetically. Meat Science, 161, 107996. https://doi.org/10.1016/j.meatsci.2019.107996

Edison, L. K., Kudva, I. T., & Kariyawasam, S. (2024). Host–Pathogen Interactions during Shiga Toxin-Producing Escherichia coli Adherence and Colonization in the Bovine Gut: A Comprehensive Review. Microorganisms, 12(10), 2009. https://doi.org/10.3390/microorganisms12102009

Knowles, T. G., Kestin, S. C., Haslam, S. M., Brown, S. N., Green, L. E., Butterworth, A., Pope, S. J., Pfeiffer, D., & Nicol, C. J. (2008). Leg disorders in broiler chickens: Prevalence, risk factors, and prevention. *PLOS ONE, 3*(2), e1545. https://doi.org/10.1371/journal.pone.0001545

Landers, T. F., Cohen, B., Wittum, T. E., & Larson, E. L. (2012). A review of antibiotic use in food animals: Perspective, policy, and potential. *Public Health Reports, 127*(1), 4–22. https://doi.org/10.1177/003335491212700103

Laxminarayan, R., Duse, A., Wattal, C., & Zaidi, A. K. M. (2013). Antibiotic resistance: The need for global solutions. *The Lancet Infectious Diseases, 13*(12), 1057–1098. https://doi.org/10.1016/S1473-3099(13)70318-9

Marchant-Forde, J. N. (Ed.). (2009). The welfare of pigs (By C. Phillips). Springer ScienceþBusiness Media B.V. https://doi.org/10.1007/978-1-4020-8909-1

Mench, J., Sumner, D., & Rosen-Molina, J. (2010). Sustainability of egg production in the United States—The policy and market context. Poultry Science, 90(1), 229–240. https://doi.org/10.3382/ps.2010-00844Oltenacu, P., & Broom, D. (2010). The impact of genetic selection for increased milk yield on the welfare of dairy cows. *Animal Welfare, 19*(S1), 39–49. https://doi.org/10.1017/S0962728600002220

Reganold, J. P., & Wachter, J. M. (2016). Organic agriculture in the twenty-first century. *Nature Plants, 2*(2), 15221. https://doi.org/10.1038/nplants.2015.221

Russell, J. B., & Rychlik, J. L. (2001). Factors that alter rumen microbial ecology. *Science, 292*(5519), 1119–1122. https://doi.org/10.1126/science.1058830

Soto, A. M., & Sonnenschein, C. (2010). Environmental causes of cancer: Endocrine disruptors as carcinogens. *Nature Reviews Endocrinology, 6*(7), 363–370. https://doi.org/10.1038/nrendo.2010.87

Vandenberg, L. N., Colborn, T., Hayes, T. B., Heindel, J. J., Jacobs, D. R., Lee, D. H., Shioda, T., Soto, A. M., vom Saal, F. S., Welshons, W. V., Zoeller, R. T., & Myers, J. P. (2012). Hormones and endocrine-disrupting chemicals: Low-dose effects and nonmonotonic dose responses. *Endocrine Reviews, 33*(3), 378–455. https://doi.org/10.1210/er.2011-1050

Most, M. S., & Yates, D. T. (2021). Inflammatory mediation of heat Stress-Induced growth Deficits in livestock and its potential role as a target for nutritional interventions: a review. Animals, 11(12), 3539. https://doi.org/10.3390/ani11123539

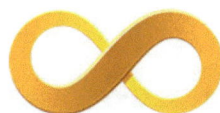

SECTION II: Physiology, Breath, and Resilience

Rewiring the Nervous System: Ancient Practices for Modern Resilience

The human nervous system can be likened to an electrical system designed for specific voltage and amperage. Traditionally, it is assumed that most individuals are wired for 110 volts and 10 amps. However, contemporary society necessitates functioning at 220 volts and 30 amps, far exceeding the capacity originally intended by our biology. This increased "voltage" manifests as chronic stress, anxiety, burnout, and various physical ailments.

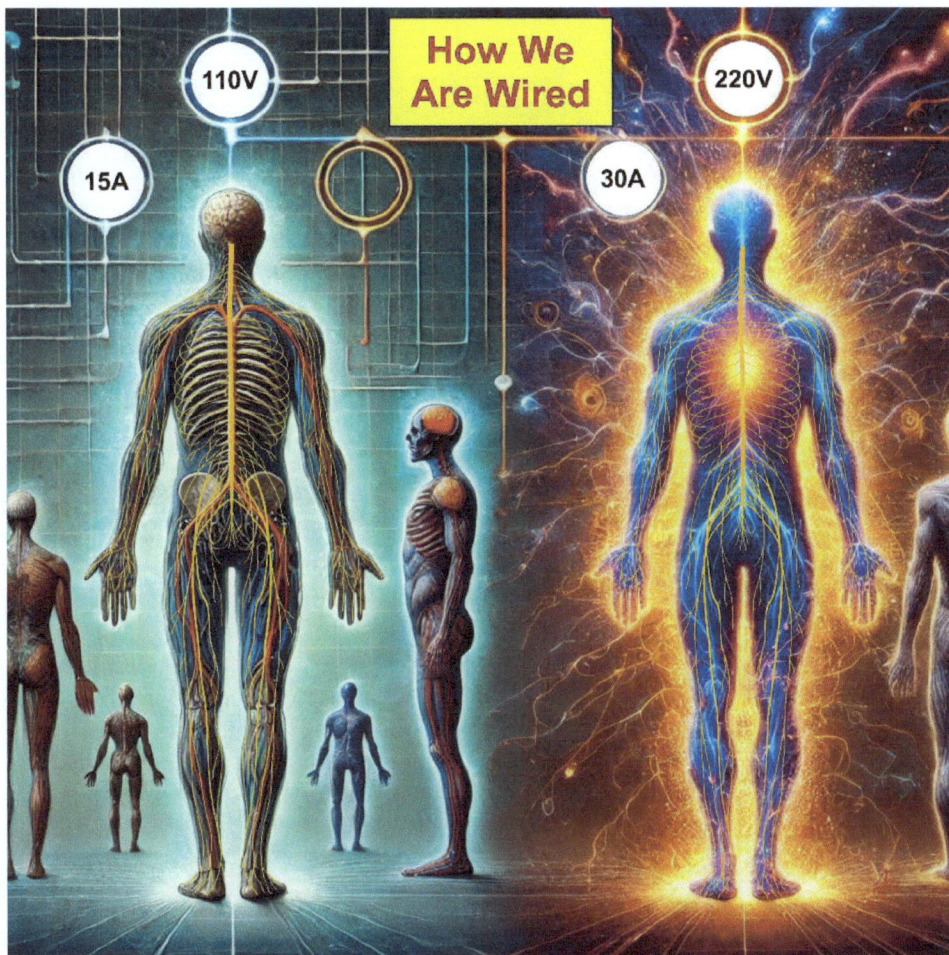

Nevertheless, just as an electrical system can be rewired to handle greater loads, the human nervous system can also be trained to adapt. Ancient practices such as martial arts, qigong, Dao Yin (Taoist yoga), yoga, and breathwork serve as effective interventions. These time-tested methods bridge the gap between the body's inherent capabilities and the demands of modern life, enabling the nervous system to withstand higher levels of stress without succumbing to being overwhelmed.

The Role of Stance Training and Controlled Stress

With over 45 years of experience in martial arts, qigong, Dao Yin, and yoga, it has been observed that certain methods can effectively enhance the nervous system. One such method is stance training, which involves holding postures for specific durations while integrating breath control.

For beginners, basic stances are introduced in succession, initially without prolonged holds. As they progress, duration gradually increases. Once students can hold each stance for 30 seconds, controlled breathing is incorporated, typically three breaths per 30 seconds. With consistent practice, the duration is extended to one-minute holds, adjusting breath cycles to around four to six respirations per minute.

This approach serves multiple purposes. On a physical level, it strengthens the legs, core, and other stabilizing muscles. On a neurological level, it encourages the nervous system to adapt to discomfort, fostering resilience, endurance, and focus. On an energetic level, it stimulates the body's internal pathways, potentially leading to enhanced vitality and internal balance.

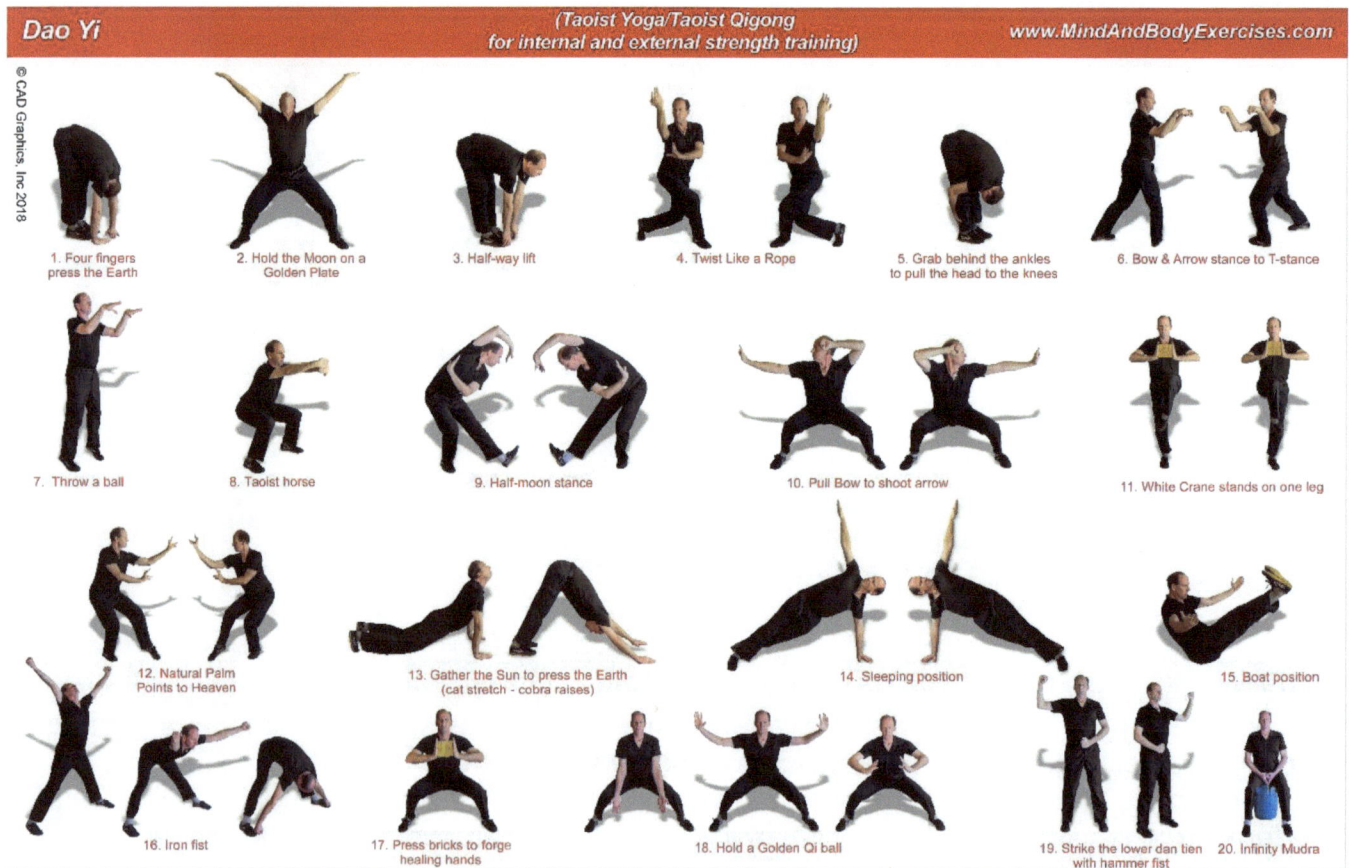

Dao Yi (Taoist Yoga/Taoist Qigong for internal and external strength training) www.MindAndBodyExercises.com

© CAD Graphics, Inc 2018

1. Four fingers press the Earth
2. Hold the Moon on a Golden Plate
3. Half-way lift
4. Twist Like a Rope
5. Grab behind the ankles to pull the head to the knees
6. Bow & Arrow stance to T-stance
7. Throw a ball
8. Taoist horse
9. Half-moon stance
10. Pull Bow to shoot arrow
11. White Crane stands on one leg
12. Natural Palm Points to Heaven
13. Gather the Sun to press the Earth (cat stretch - cobra raises)
14. Sleeping position
15. Boat position
16. Iron fist
17. Press bricks to forge healing hands
18. Hold a Golden Qi ball
19. Strike the lower dan tien with hammer fist
20. Infinity Mudra

The Science Behind the Training: The Anterior Midcingulate Cortex (aMCC)
While these practices have been in use for centuries, contemporary neuroscience provides insight into their effectiveness. A critical region of the brain implicated in resilience is the anterior midcingulate cortex (aMCC).

The aMCC is responsible for effortful control, emotional regulation, and persistence in the face of challenges. Research indicates that engaging in controlled stress—such as maintaining difficult stances, regulating breath, or training under discomfort—strengthens and enlarging the aMCC. Consequently, individuals who practice these methods may enhance their ability to manage stress more effectively, increase mental toughness, and maintain composure under pressure.

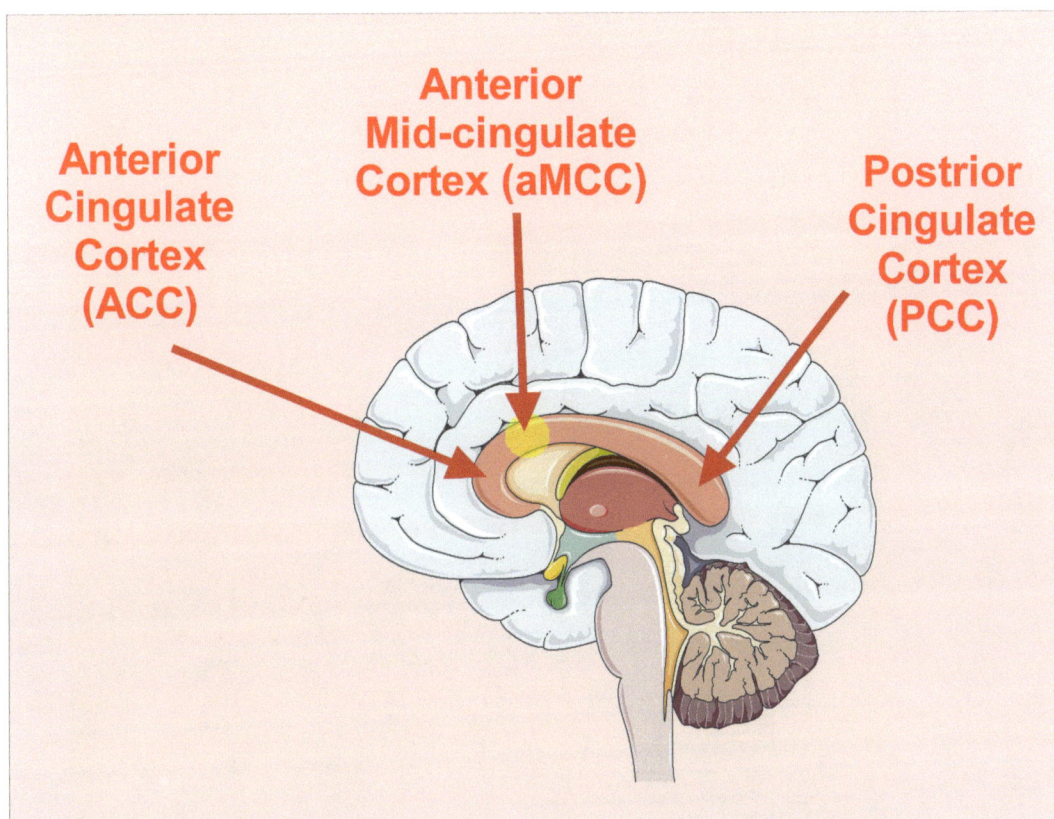

In essence, deliberate training can augment our capacity to handle life's challenges, analogous to how lifting heavier weights strengthens muscles. This concept is consistent with the principle of progressive overload, which is well-established in strength training and equally applicable to the nervous system and mental resilience.

"Burning the *Chong Mai*" – The Energetic Dimension

Beyond the physical and neurological aspects, these practices have deep roots in Taoist and Traditional Chinese Medicine (TCM). An important concept in energetic cultivation is "burning the Chong Mai."

The Chong Mai (Thrusting Vessel) is one of the eight extraordinary meridians in TCM. It serves as a primary channel for deep energy reserves, influencing the body's overall energy flow. When stance work and controlled breathing are practiced regularly, this meridian can be activated, which may allow for greater energy circulation through the other seven extraordinary vessels and the twelve main meridians.

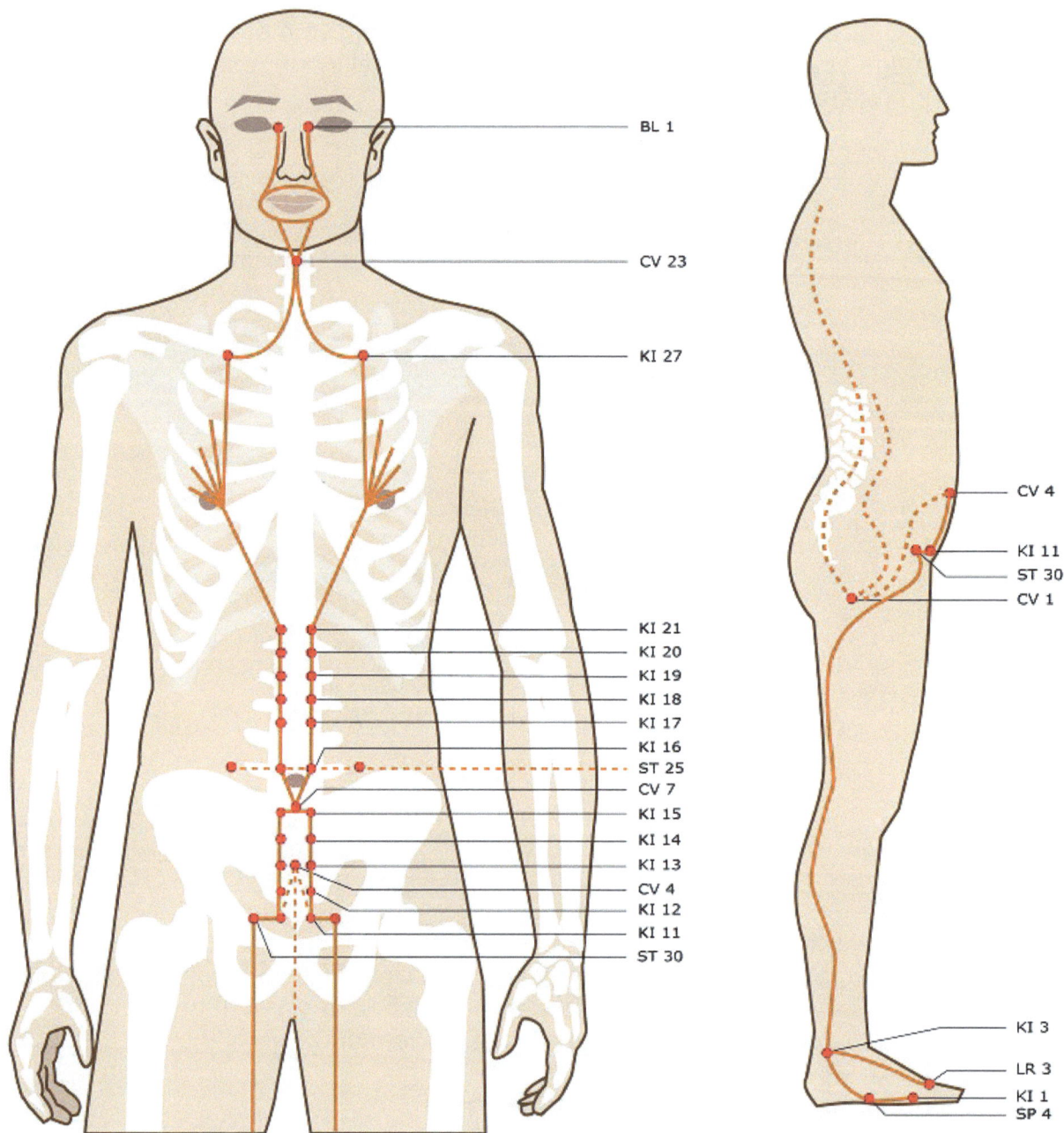

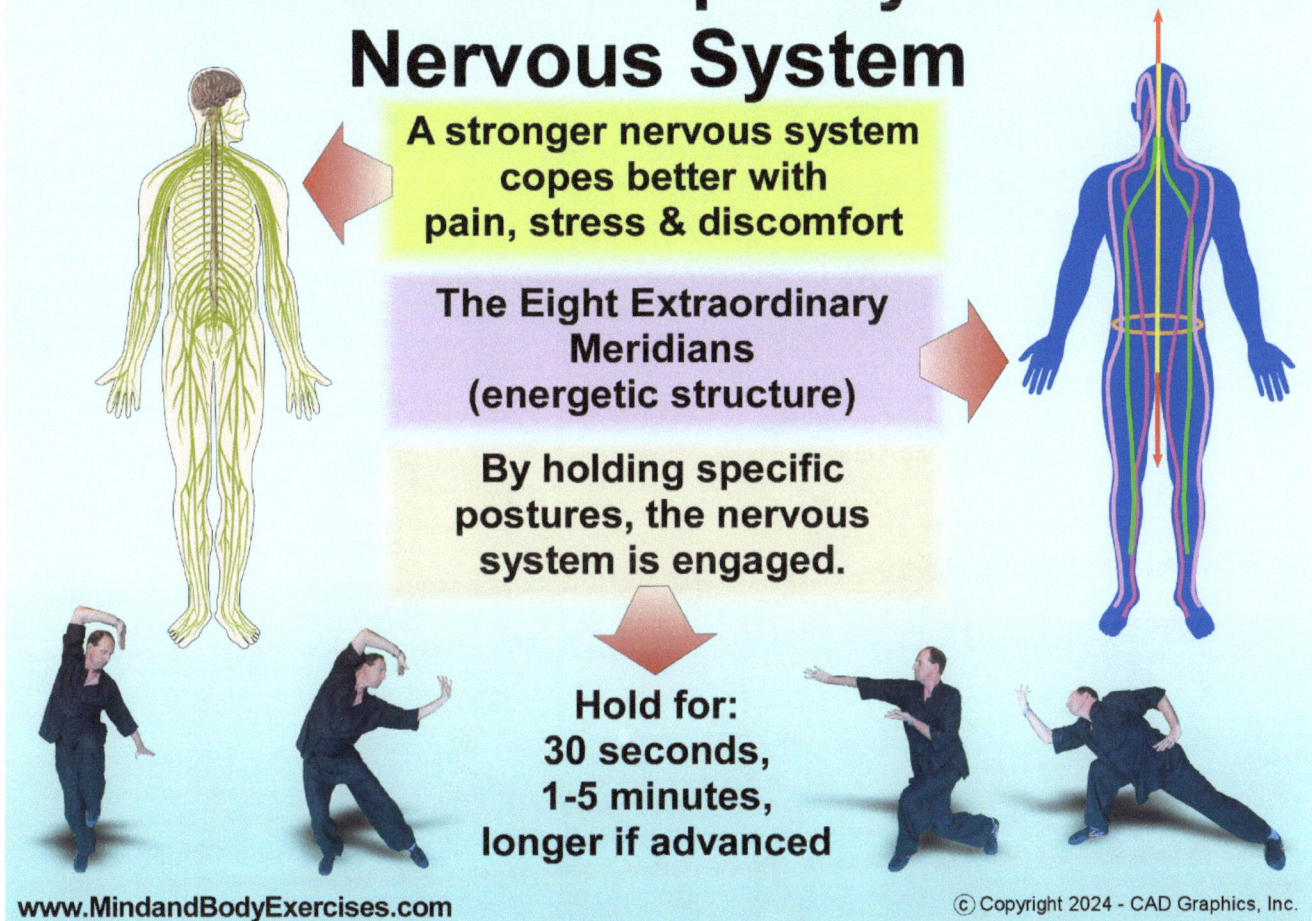

Increase the Capacity of Your Nervous System

A stronger nervous system copes better with pain, stress & discomfort

The Eight Extraordinary Meridians (energetic structure)

By holding specific postures, the nervous system is engaged.

Hold for:
30 seconds,
1-5 minutes,
longer if advanced

www.MindandBodyExercises.com

© Copyright 2024 - CAD Graphics, Inc.

This process can be compared to upgrading a power grid. By increasing the capacity of the Chong Mai, the entire energetic system can become more efficient, stable, and resilient. This observation might explain why long-term practitioners of qigong, Dao Yin, and martial arts often report higher energy levels, improved focus, and a significant sense of internal strength.

Resilience Through Discomfort: The Path to Transformation

The old adage *"That which does not kill us makes us stronger"* perfectly encapsulates the philosophy behind these training methods. Rather than avoiding stress, we use it as a tool for growth.

- **Physically**, stance training builds strength, endurance, and structural integrity.

- **Mentally**, breath control and effortful posture-holding train the nervous system to remain calm under pressure.

- **Neurologically**, the aMCC adapts and strengthens, improving stress management and persistence.

35

- **Energetically**, activating the Chong Mai and meridian system enhances internal power and resilience.

Instead of being overwhelmed by modern life's "220 volts," we can upgrade our own internal wiring, ensuring that we remain grounded, adaptive, and powerful in an ever-changing world. For those seeking true strength—not just physically, but mentally and spiritually—these ancient methods offer a proven path to transformation. The key is consistency, patience, and a willingness to embrace discomfort as a gateway to resilience.

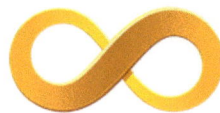

Sleep Deprivation

Sleep is a natural regularly occurring physiological function, where humans and other animals reduce physical and mental activity, lessen responsiveness to stimuli, and particular patterns of brain activity occur (Ettinger 2018). Prolonged lack of sleep or sleep deprivation can cause impaired memory formation as well as adverse effects on the brain's other cognitive functions such as learning, language, reason, and perception. Sleep deprivation has also been linked to significant mental diseases, such as depression, psychosis, and bipolar disorder (Horowitz, 2020). Physical problems attributed to consistent lack of sleep include weakening of the immune system, headaches, heart disease, fainting, weight gain or weight loss, blurred vision, and hernias. Other related ailments may include obesity, cancer, stroke, asthma, high blood pressure, diabetes, arthritis, and kidney failure. Severe sleep deprivation in humans can also be fatal, where a rare neurological ailment called fatal familial insomnia results in damage to areas of the thalamus
(Horowitz, 2020).

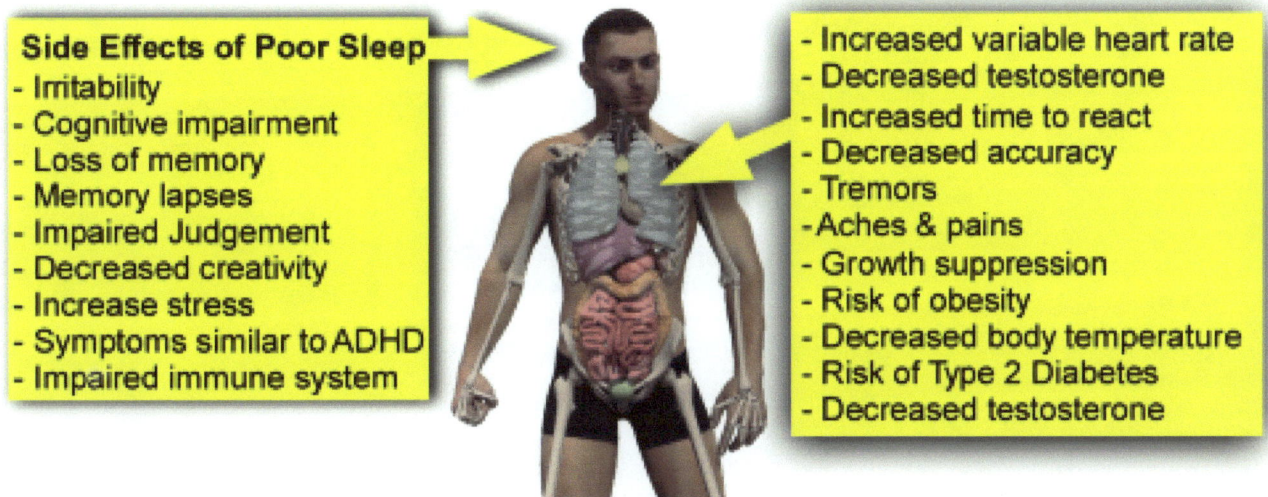

Side Effects of Poor Sleep
- Irritability
- Cognitive impairment
- Loss of memory
- Memory lapses
- Impaired Judgement
- Decreased creativity
- Increase stress
- Symptoms similar to ADHD
- Impaired immune system

- Increased variable heart rate
- Decreased testosterone
- Increased time to react
- Decreased accuracy
- Tremors
- Aches & pains
- Growth suppression
- Risk of obesity
- Decreased body temperature
- Risk of Type 2 Diabetes
- Decreased testosterone

© Copyright 2020 - CAD Graphics, Inc.

Studies with REM-deprived sleep participants showed the effects of decreased ability to concentrate on tasks, increased irritability, hostility, anxiousness, and aggressiveness. Studies also showed that REM-starved participants entered into REM sleep almost as soon as they were permitted to nod off, over the course of a one-week experiment. Participants experienced a REM rebound effect, where they spent roughly 50 percent more time in REM than they did before the start of the experiment. This REM rebound effect seems to occur immediately after a duration of forced wakefulness during a night's sleep. Physiological changes in animals have been observed in other studies regarding REM deprivation, with effects of weight loss, deteriorated appearance, skin lesions, increased energy expenditure, decreased body temperature, and even death. Researchers think that if humans experienced similar circumstances of sleep deprivation used in animal studies, similar outcomes would present (Ettinger 2018).

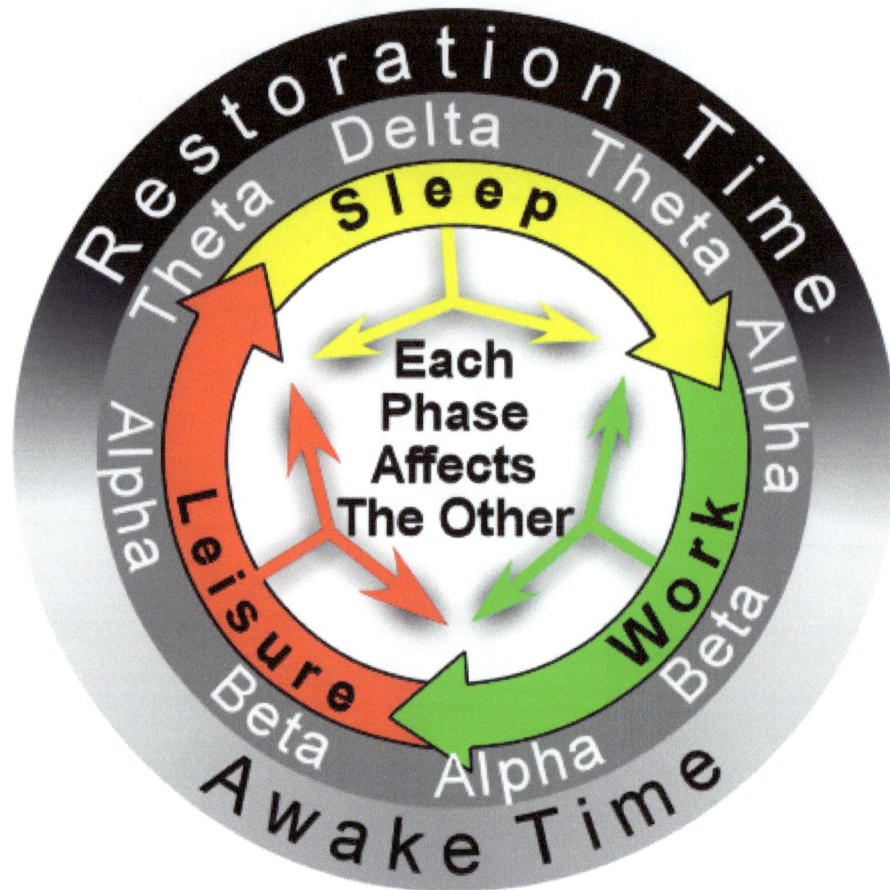

© Copyright 2020 - CAD Graphics, Inc.

Studies show that sleep is necessary, but exactly why is not clear. Theories exist that we require sleep to conserve energy, avoid predation, and memory aid. However, none of these theories are widely accepted by psychologists. Another theory is that sleep helps in mental and physical restoration. Sleep is thought to restore resources that are drained during our daily activities. Studies show that people often sleep longer after particularly tiring events help to support this theory. Unsettled evidence shows that specific types of tissue restoration might happen during sleep. Growth hormone is secreted at increased levels during Stage 4 sleep as well as brain neurotransmitters possibly being restored during sleep. Other research indicates that sleep is essential for brain homeostasis. Additionally, research suggests that metabolic waste that accumulates from neural activity is eliminated from the brain and cerebral spinal fluid, while only occurring during sleep (Ettinger 2018). This theory has merit, as other relative studies offer further evidence of sleep quality affecting health and well-being, specifically with intensive care unit (ICU) patients (Pisani, 2015). I find it hard to discredit this theory, just based on personal experience with almost everyone I have ever known or met, expressing how much more restored, refreshed, and energetic they are when they have regular quality sleep.

AGE GROUP	RECOMMENDED HOURS OF SLEEP
Newborns (0-3 months)	14-17 hours
Infants (4-11 months)	12-15 hours
Toddlers (1-2 years)	11-14 hours
Pre-Schoolers (3-5 years)	10-13 hours
School Age (6-12 years)	9-11 hours
Teenagers (13-17 years)	8-10 hours
Young Adults (18-25 years)	7-9 hours
Adults (26-64 years)	7-9 hours
Seniors (65 & older)	7-8 hours

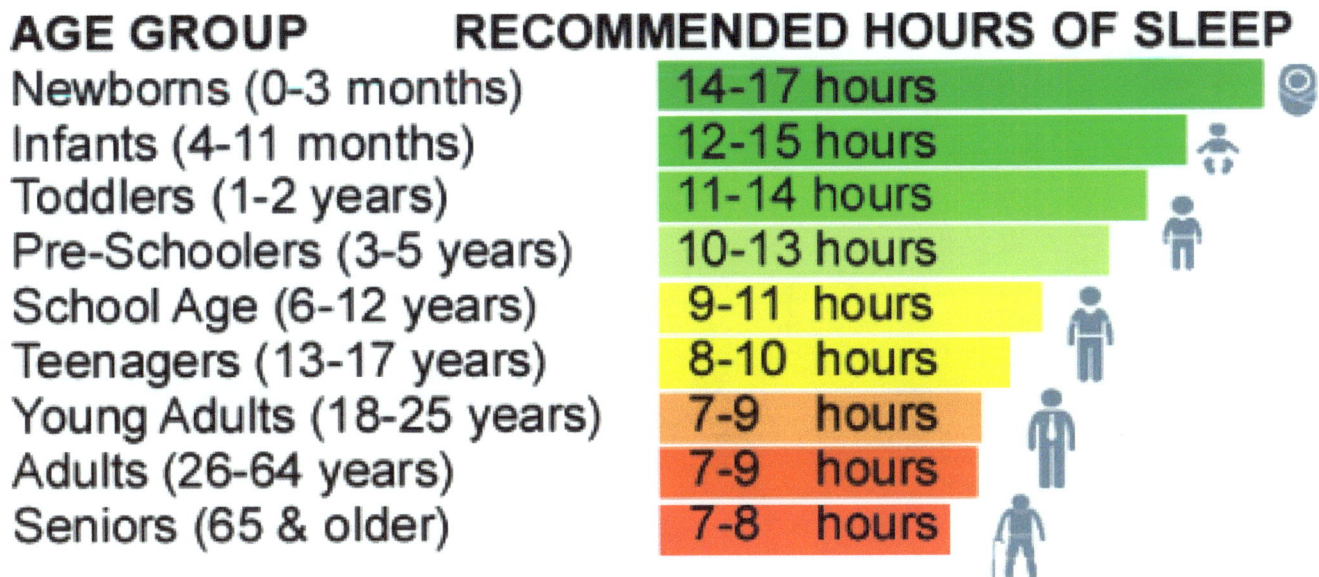

© Copyright 2020 - CAD Graphics, Inc.

I feel that American culture in general, does not pay much attention to preventing disease and illness, let alone the specific issue of sleep deprivation. We have gradually grown into a nation where we live for our pleasures today, with little regard for the consequences that will come tomorrow. Many see modern allopathic medicine and its many pharmaceutical options as the only path to fixing all of our ills. There is a plethora of medications that we can take to keep us awake when we don't get enough sleep. Conversely, we also have a wide variety of other pharmaceuticals to help us sleep when we are too awake, anxious, or stressed.

I see many college-aged kids, who are learning how to manage and navigate their college lives of studies and social life, while also trying to stay safe and healthy in the process. I don't really think the issue of college student sleep deprivation has changed much over the last few decades, as far as young adults exercising their independence and learning of their limits. What has changed, I believe is the acceptance of legal as well as illegal drugs being used to manage the ups and downs of coping with the on-campus "college life". Additionally, the last 2 years of dealing with the COVID-19 pandemic have greatly added to the recipe for potential psychological issues. Many people of all ages have experienced stress as they attempt to balance their relative circumstances. Many people were inside more which may have led to a more sedentary lifestyle, eating more poor-quality food, drinking more alcohol, consuming more recreation and medicinal drugs, and other issues that can affect the quality of sleep. Consequently, I think the more relative issue that is yet to unfold, is how has the management of the pandemic affected sleep quality across many demographics? This topic will probably take years to study in order to draw any logical conclusions.

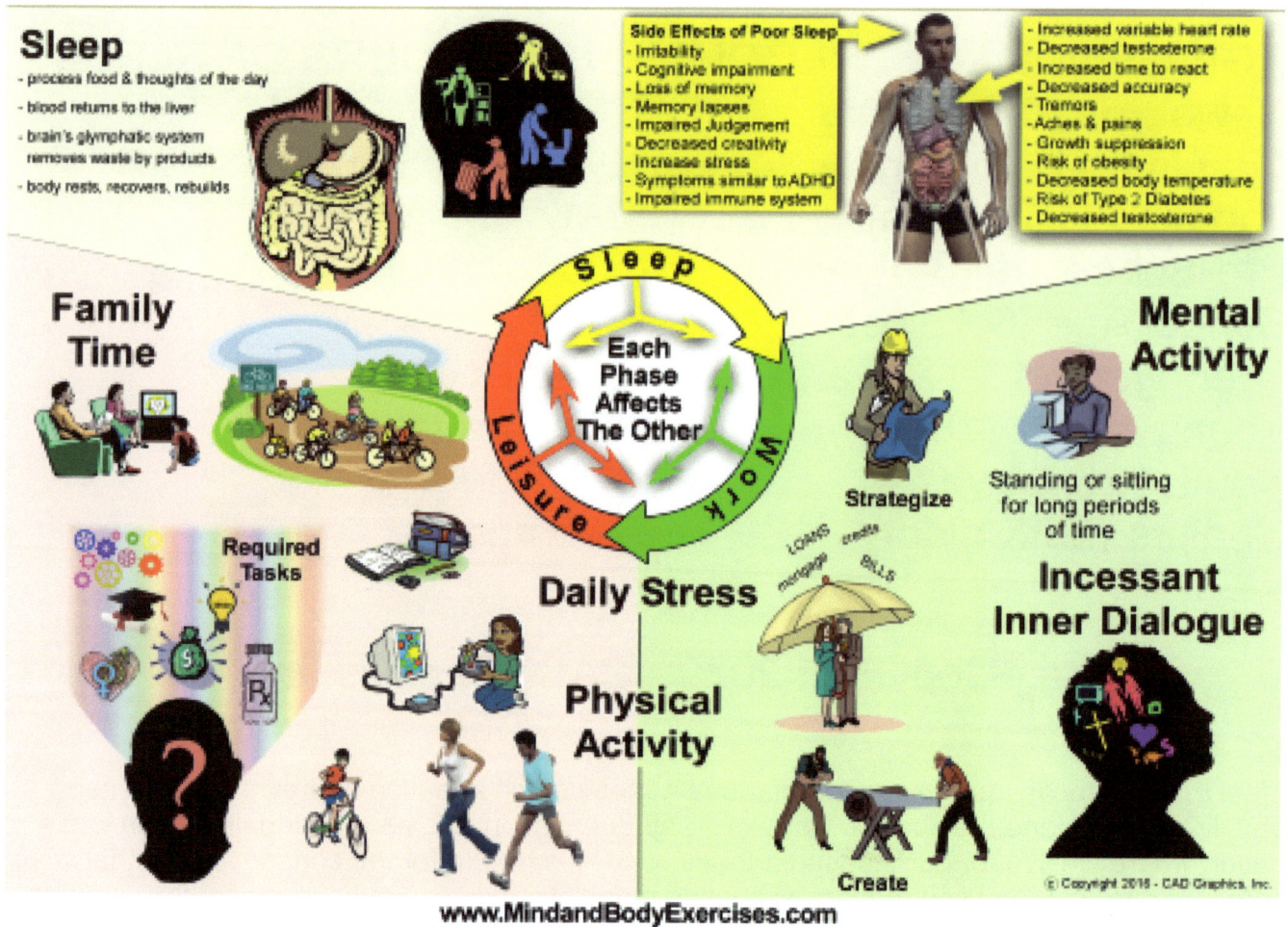

References:

Ettinger, R. H. (2018). Psychology: The Science of Behavior (6th ed.). BVT Publishing.
Horowitz, D. (2020). Sleep deprivation. Salem Press Encyclopedia of Health.

Pisani, M. (2015). Sleep in the intensive care unit: An oft-neglected key to health restoration.

Heart & Lung : The Journal of Critical Care, 44(2), 87. https://doi-org.northernvermont.idm.oclc.org/10.1016/j.hrtlng.2015.01.007

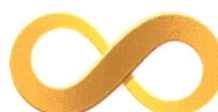

Primary Muscles Used in Respiration

Breathing is supported by a complex system of muscles, with the diaphragm and intercostals playing primary roles in quiet, relaxed breathing, while accessory muscles like the SCM, scalenes, and pectoralis minor assist during times of physical exertion or respiratory distress. Maintaining balanced breathing patterns focused on diaphragmatic and nasal breathing minimizes tension in the neck, shoulders, and chest, promoting relaxation and better oxygenation. Understanding and nurturing this system can enhance respiratory health, reduce muscle tension, and improve overall well-being.

Muscles of Inspiration

CORE MUSCLES

- external intercostal
(contracts to elevate ribs)

- diaphragm
(contracts to expand thoracic cavity)

ACCESSORY MUSCLES

- sternocleidomastoid
(contracts to elevate sternum)

- pectoralis minor
(contracts to pull ribs outwards)

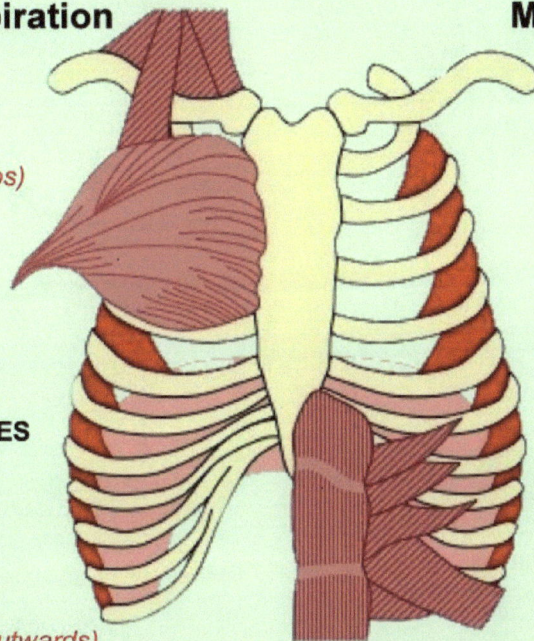

Muscles of Expiration

CORE MUSCLES

- internal intercostal
(contracts to pull ribs down)

- diaphragm
(relaxes to reduce thoracic cavity)

ACCESSORY MUSCLES

- abdominals
(contracts to compress abdomen)

- quadratus lumborum
(contracts to pull ribs down)

www.MindAndBodyExercises.com

© Copyright 2025 - CAD Graphics, Inc.

The Mechanics of Breathing: An In-Depth Look at Respiratory Muscles

Breathing involves various muscles throughout the body, working together to facilitate the intake of oxygen and the expulsion of carbon dioxide. This process is orchestrated by different muscle groups that support both relaxed respiration and the increased demands of exercise or stress. This article examines the primary and accessory muscles involved in breathing, including the diaphragm, neck, and chest muscles, and analyzes their contribution to respiratory efficiency and posture.

Primary Muscles of Respiration

The diaphragm plays a crucial role in respiration, accounting for approximately 75% of the effort during relaxed or "tidal" breathing. Situated below the lungs and above the abdominal cavity, this dome-shaped muscle contracts and flattens downward with each inhalation, creating negative pressure within the thoracic cavity and allowing air to enter the lungs. Upon exhalation, the diaphragm relaxes and returns to its dome shape, gently pushing air out as the lungs recoil. Efficient diaphragmatic function is essential for relaxed breathing and overall respiratory health, particularly when breathing through the nose.

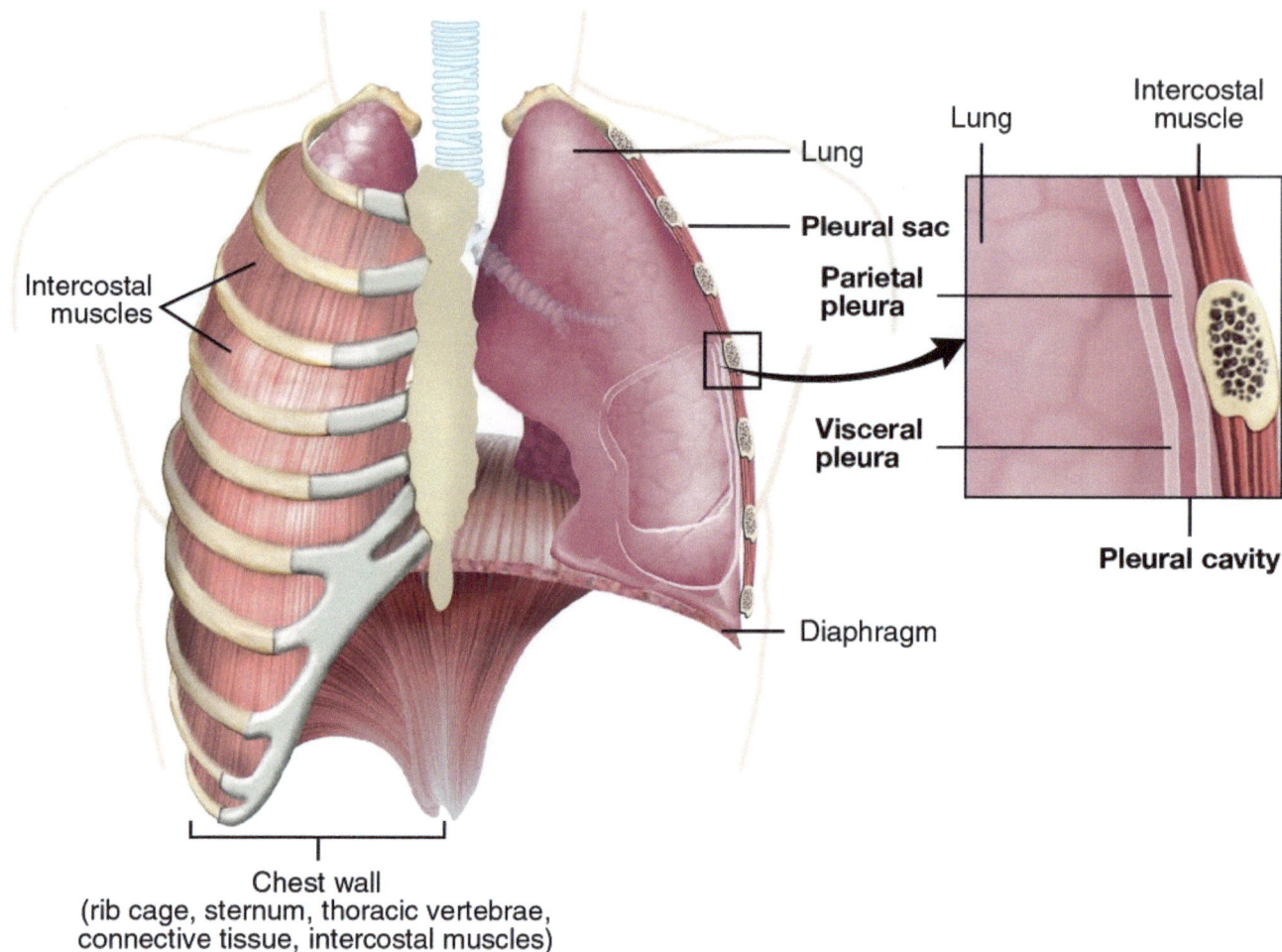

Chest wall
(rib cage, sternum, thoracic vertebrae,
connective tissue, intercostal muscles)

The intercostal muscles work in conjunction with the diaphragm to expand and contract the rib cage, supporting respiration. Located between the ribs, these muscles are divided into two groups:

External intercostals, which are primarily active during inhalation, lift the rib cage up and outward, expanding the chest cavity and allowing more air into the lungs.

Internal intercostals, which are mainly involved during forced exhalation, pull the rib cage down and inward, compressing the chest to expel air forcefully.

Together, the diaphragm and intercostals comprise the primary muscles of breathing, efficiently managing inhalation and exhalation during quiet respiration without requiring assistance from other muscles. The costovertebral joints and sternocostal joints are important for respiration by enabling the movement of the rib cage during breathing.

Costovertebral Joints: These are the articulations between the ribs and the thoracic vertebrae. Each rib connects to the vertebral column at two points—the costovertebral joint (where the rib meets the vertebral body) and the costotransverse joint (where the rib meets the transverse process of the vertebra). These joints allow the ribs to move in a pump-handle (expanding the chest upward) and bucket-handle (widening the chest laterally) motion, which increases the volume of the thoracic cavity during inhalation.

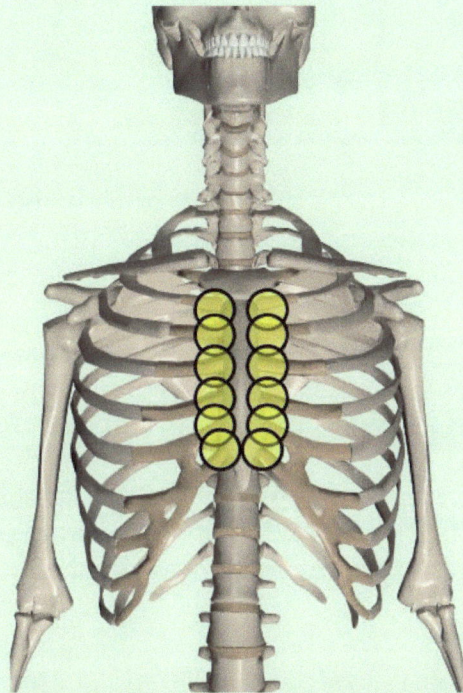

Sternocostal Joints: These are the connections between the ribs and the sternum. The first rib forms a direct synchondrosis (cartilaginous joint) with the sternum, while ribs 2–7 have synovial joints that allow for slight gliding movements. These joints enable the sternum to elevate and expand along with rib movement, assisting in lung expansion.

Joints of the Rib Cage That Affect Breathing

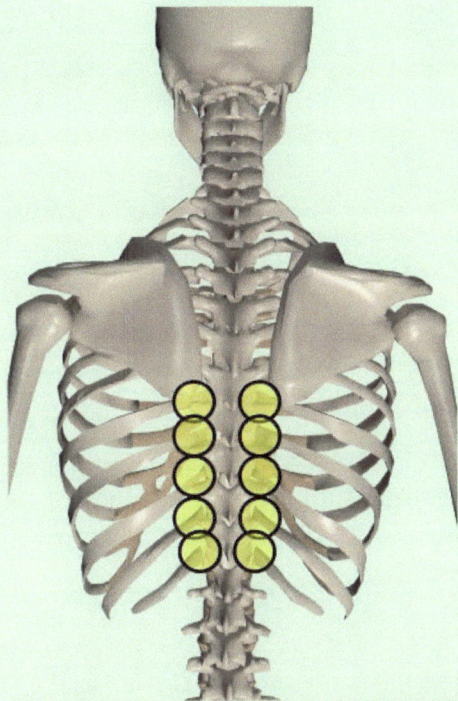

costal vertebral joints   sternocostal joints

www.MindAndBodyExercises.com　　　　　　　　　　　　　　　ⓒ Copyright 2025 - CAD Graphics, Inc.

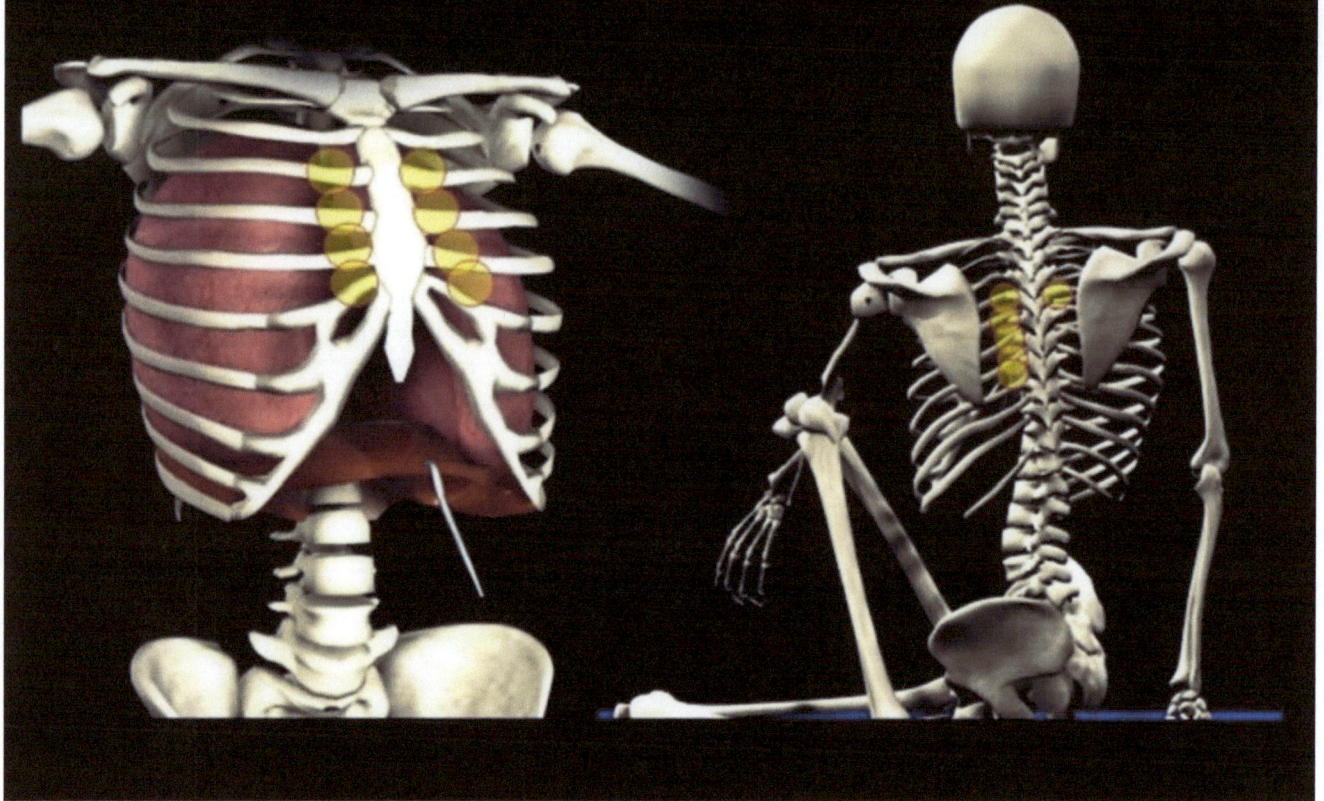

Effect of vertebral Rotation on Respiratory Functions

Together, these joints provide flexibility and stability to the rib cage, supporting efficient breathing by accommodating the expansion and contraction required for proper lung function. Issues or stiffness in these joints can restrict breathing efficiency and contribute to postural problems.

The Role of Accessory Muscles in Breathing

During labored breathing, such as physical exertion, illness, or stress, additional muscles assist the diaphragm and intercostals in expanding and contracting the rib cage and chest. These accessory muscles of respiration include:

Sternocleidomastoid (SCM) and scalene muscles in the neck are particularly important accessory muscles. The SCM connects the base of the skull to the sternum and clavicle, helping lift the sternum and clavicle during inhalation to expand the upper chest. Similarly, the scalenes (anterior, middle, and posterior) attach from the cervical vertebrae to the first two ribs, assisting in lifting the upper chest and creating additional space in the lungs. During high-effort breathing, these muscles help maximize airflow but can lead to neck tension if overused, especially in those with shallow breathing patterns.

The pectoralis minor, located beneath the larger pectoralis major in the upper chest, attaches from the ribs to the scapula (shoulder blade). During forced inhalation, it helps lift the upper ribs, expanding the chest cavity.

The serratus anterior also supports respiration, particularly during heavy breathing. Attached to the ribs and scapula, it stabilizes the upper chest, allowing greater lung expansion. While effective in aiding respiration, overuse of the pectoralis minor and serratus anterior can cause tightness in the chest and shoulders, contributing to poor posture and reduced respiratory efficiency.

Nasal Breathing vs. Mouth Breathing

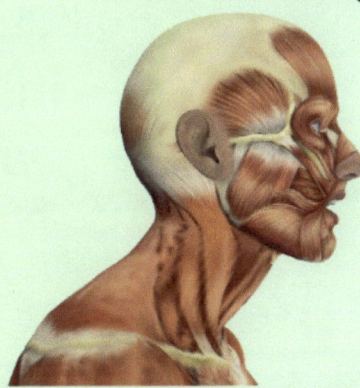

Among many healthcare professionals, fitness enthusiasts, martial artists, musical instrument performers, and others understand that breathing through the nose, or nasal breathing is generally considered better than breathing solely through the mouth for several reasons.

Nasal Breathing

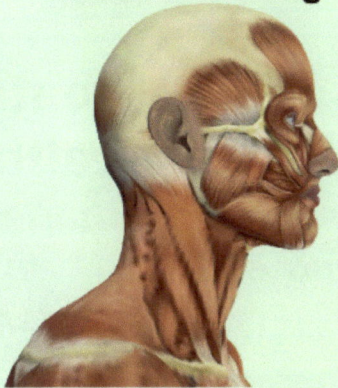

- Filters dust, allergens, and pathogens
- Enhances oxygen absorption
- Humidifies and warms incoming air
- Produces nitric oxide (boosts circulation & immunity)
- Encourages deep, diaphragmatic breathing
- Improves sleep quality (reduces snoring & apnea)
- Prevents dry mouth, reducing oral health issues
- Increases endurance and athletic performance
- Maintains proper CO2-O2 balance for calmness
- Supports proper facial and jaw development
- Reduces stress and anxiety
- Enhances cognitive function and focus
- Supports good posture and tongue placement
- Improves voice quality and resonance

Mouth Breathing

- Allows unfiltered air, increasing allergen exposure
- Reduces oxygen efficiency
- Dries out the mouth, leading to cavities & gum disease
- Increases risk of respiratory infections
- Disrupts sleep (linked to snoring & sleep apnea)
- Lowers nitric oxide production, affecting circulation
- Can cause poor facial development in children
- Leads to shallow breathing and poor posture
- Raises stress levels and contributes to anxiety
- Reduces endurance and physical performance
- Can weaken immune function
- May cause speech and vocal issues

www.MindAndBodyExercises.com

Other accessory muscles include the levator scapulae and upper trapezius, which elevate and stabilize the shoulders and engage in upper chest breathing in response to stress or poor posture. Although not intended specifically for breathing, these muscles often become involved when the diaphragm is not fully engaged, potentially leading to chronic tension in the neck and upper back.

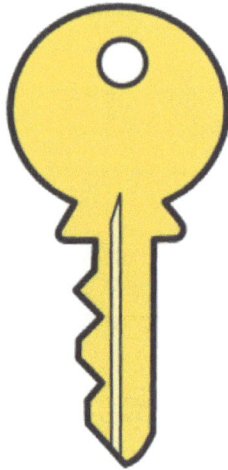

The quality of the breath, determines the quality of one's health

most see the breath like on or off, with little in between.
"If you're breathing, you're good!"

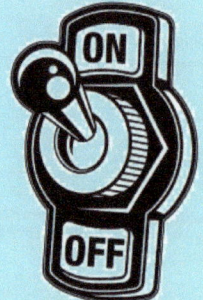

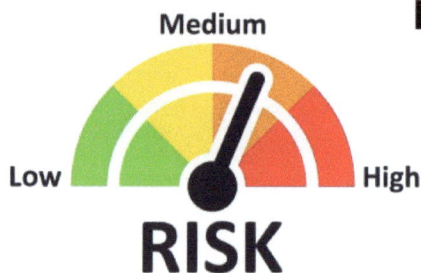

instead, try to see the breath as a gauge to better health.
Slow and deep breathing, manages stress and emotions and consequently, the nervous system

Medium

Low   High

RISK

The Role of Abdominal Muscles and Core Stabilizers

The abdominal muscles, including the rectus abdominis, transversus abdominis, and obliques, play essential roles in forceful exhalation by increasing abdominal pressure and pushing the diaphragm up, expelling air during activities such as coughing, singing, or exercising. While these muscles do not contribute to inhalation during quiet breathing, strong abdominal muscles support core stability and posture, indirectly promoting efficient diaphragm function.

Smaller, deeper muscles like the multifidus and deep cervical flexors support posture and spinal alignment, ensuring that the rib cage can expand without restriction. These muscles

46

indirectly contribute to breathing by maintaining good posture, reducing unnecessary tension, and keeping the airway open.

Implications of Respiratory Muscle Engagement on Health and Posture

Efficient breathing relies on primary respiratory muscles, with the diaphragm and intercostals as key players. When these muscles are effectively engaged, the body maintains a relaxed, steady respiratory rhythm, promoting effective oxygenation and minimizing muscle tension in the neck and shoulders. Nasal breathing encourages diaphragmatic engagement, stimulating the parasympathetic nervous system and promoting relaxation.

However, many individuals develop shallow, chest-driven breathing patterns due to stress, poor posture, or habits like mouth breathing, which lead to over-reliance on accessory muscles and result in chronic neck, shoulder, and upper chest tension. Shallow breathing also activates the sympathetic nervous system, exacerbating stress and creating a cycle of inefficient respiration and muscular strain.

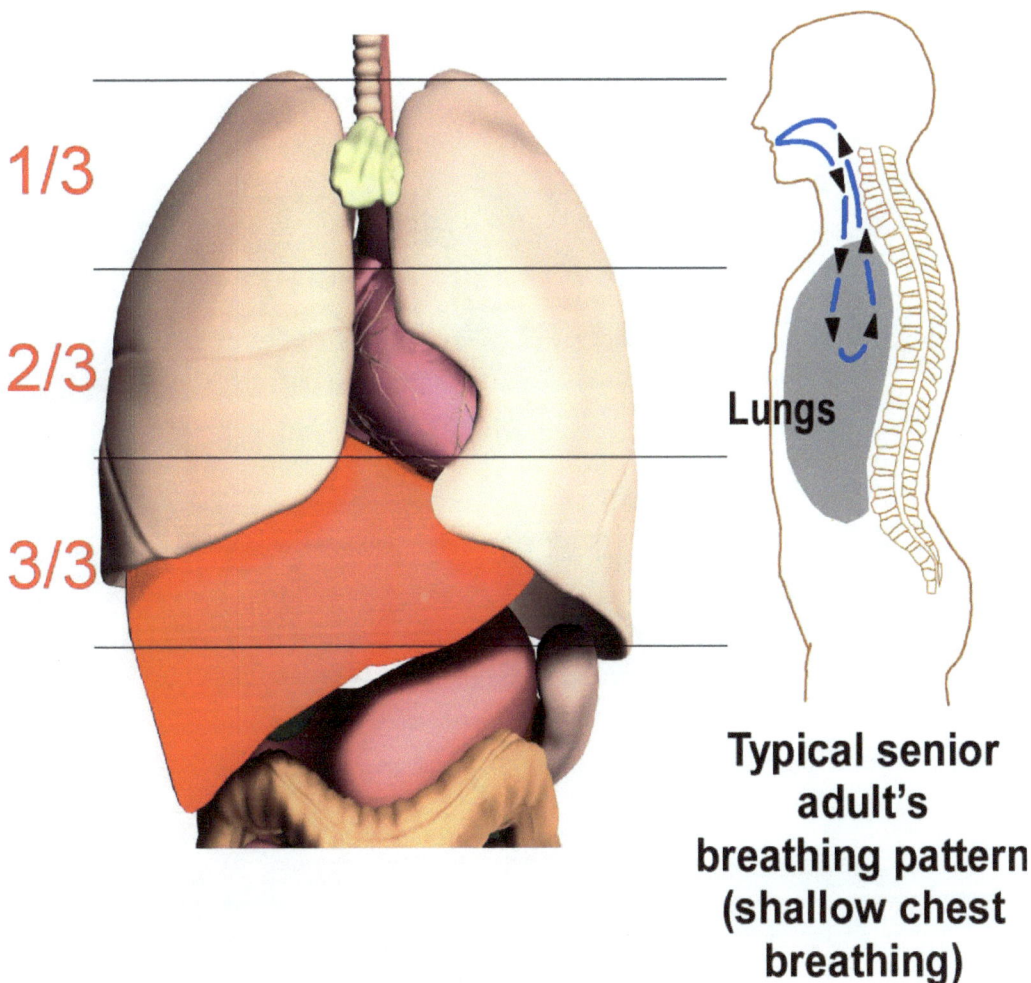

1/3
2/3
3/3

Lungs

Typical senior adult's breathing pattern (shallow chest breathing)

www.MindandBodyExercises.com

The Influence of Breath-Centered Movement Practices

Exercise methods like yoga, tai chi, qigong, and martial arts use breathing techniques to optimize respiration and lung function. They focus on deep diaphragmatic breathing paired with slow, controlled movements, such as torso twists, to stretch the intercostal and oblique muscles, expand lung capacity, and fully engage the diaphragm. Practitioners often report increased energy or transformation, with physiological benefits including optimized oxygen intake, reduced tension, and improved respiratory efficiency. These practices promote nasal breathing, effective diaphragm engagement, and a balanced autonomic nervous system, leading to better respiratory health and less stress.

Deep Breathing Benefits

Deeper breathing is a key component to having a long and healthy life. Through focused and deliberate breathing methods, many positive mental and physical benefits can be achieved.

- Diaphragm breathing acts as a pump to massage internal organs

- Movement of the diaphragm helps push lymph throughout your body, eliminating toxins while strengthening the immune system

- Improves blood circulation which oxygenates cells

- Activates the Parasympathetic Nervous System

- C02 waste is eliminated directly through the breath

Abdominal Breathing

Inhale   Exhale

Focus of awareness upon inhalation

Focus of awareness upon exhalation

Abdominal movement while breathing dramatically increases lung capacity

Inhalation: abdomen expands, diaphragm descends

Exhalation: lower abdomen is retracted, diaphragm raises

www.MindandBodyExercises.com

48

Conclusion

Breathing is supported by a complex system of muscles, with the diaphragm and intercostals playing primary roles in quiet, relaxed breathing, while accessory muscles like the SCM, scalenes, and pectoralis minor assist during times of physical exertion or respiratory distress. Maintaining balanced breathing patterns focused on diaphragmatic and nasal breathing minimizes tension in the neck, shoulders, and chest, promoting relaxation and better oxygenation. Understanding and nurturing this system can enhance respiratory health, reduce muscle tension, and improve overall well-being.

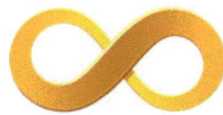

Spring Has Sprung. Are You a Wood Element Constitution?

"Knowing others is intelligence.
Knowing yourself is true wisdom.
Mastering others is strength.
Mastering yourself is true power."
— Lao Tzu, Tao Te Ching

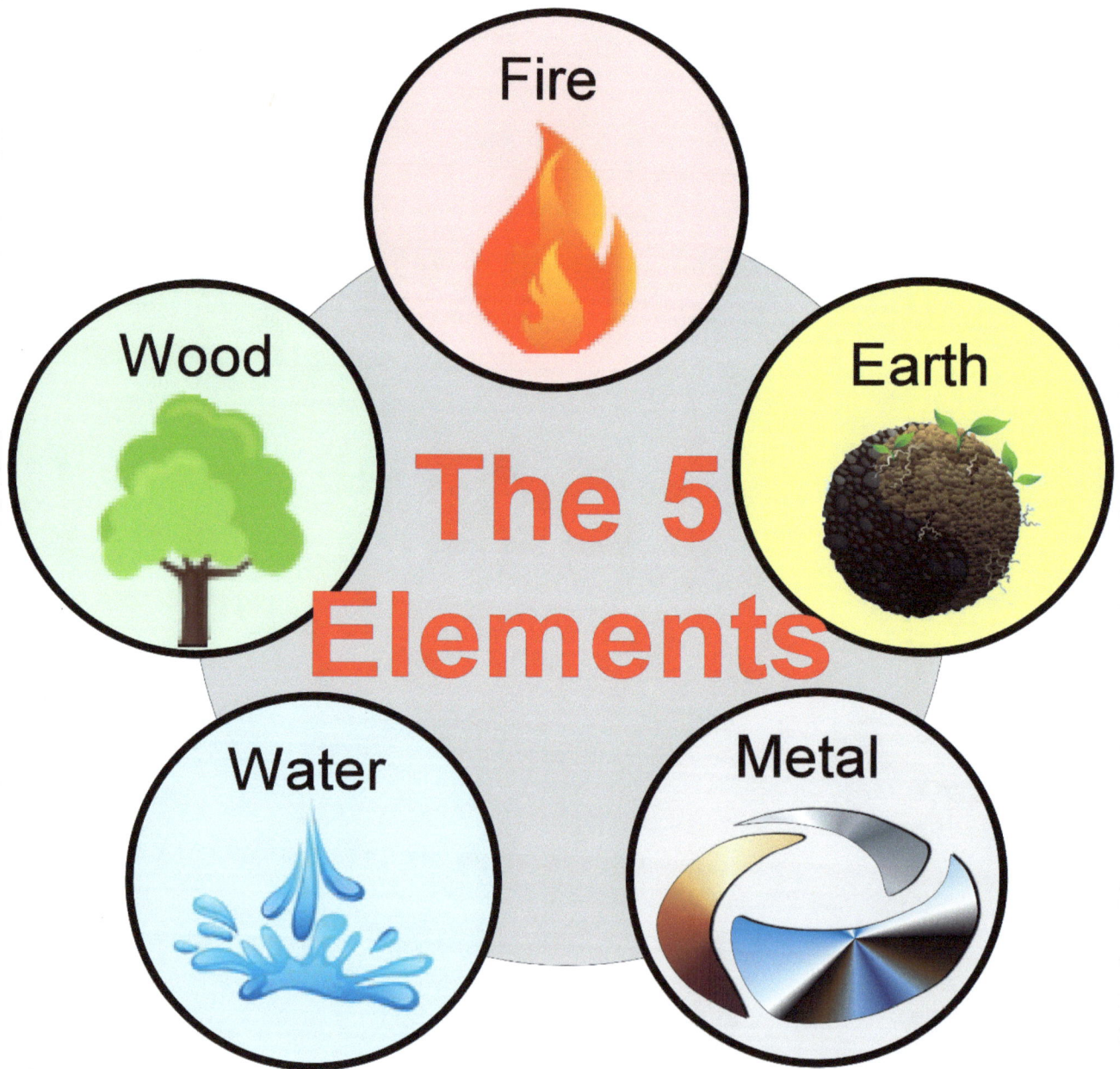

Fire

Wood

Earth

The 5 Elements

Water

Metal

Knowing one's own constitution, as well as others in their life can help to better understand how and why people behave the way they do under certain situations. Some may see this concept as somewhat controversial or as a version of "profiling." However, this concept has been used for over thousands of years in various cultures across the world, such as with Traditional Chinese Medicine (the 5 Elements), Hippocratic & Greco-Roman Medicine (the Four Humors), Jungian Psychology, Tibetan Medicine (Sowa Rigpa), Western Biopsychological Models (Sheldon's Somatotypes). Ayurveda (Indian "study of life") and indigenous peoples across the globe.

The Wood Element in Traditional Chinese Medicine

In Traditional Chinese Medicine (TCM), the Wood Element is one of the five fundamental forces in the Five Element Theory, which explains the interconnection between natural phenomena and human life. Each element of Wood, Fire, Earth, Metal, and Water corresponds to seasons of the year, specific organs, emotions, and physiological processes. Wood, in particular, is linked to the season of spring, the liver and gallbladder, shaping both physical and psychological characteristics in individuals with a "Wood constitution." The Wood Element is characterized by physical movement, ambition, and outward energy. While Wood types are dynamic and goal-driven, they must cultivate mental and physical flexibility, and adequate rest to prevent stress and stagnation.

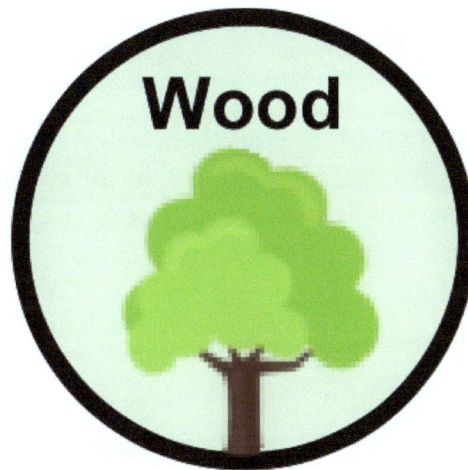

1. **Physical Traits of a Wood Constitution**

   - **Body Structure:** Individuals influenced by the Wood Element typically have a sinewy, muscular build, often appearing strong and tall with an inherent sense of vitality.

   - **Strength and Flexibility:** They usually possess endurance and adaptability, both physically and mentally, with a natural propensity toward movement and expansion.

- **Common Health Challenges:** Wood types may encounter liver and/or gallbladder-related concerns, including digestive disturbances, migraines, muscle and tendon stiffness, and detoxification difficulties. Liver Qi stagnation can also lead to menstrual irregularities or eye discomfort.

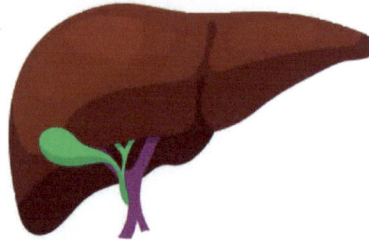

Positive	Negative
Kindness	Anger
Generosity	Jealousy
	Envy

2. Mental and Emotional Aspects

- **Core Emotion:** The primary emotion linked to Wood is anger. When balanced, Wood individuals express healthy assertiveness, confidence, and determination. However, an imbalance can lead to frustration, irritability or struggles with managing emotions.

- **Personality and Leadership:** Wood types are often natural leaders, driven by vision, ambition, and a desire for growth. They excel in planning and organization, where they always seek progress.

- **Decision-Making:** They tend to be quite decisive and pioneering, eager to initiate change.

- **Emotional Imbalances:** When unbalanced, Wood individuals may become uptight, rigid, impatient, overly perfectionistic, and prone to burnout from excessive effort.

3. Spiritual Dimensions
- **Growth and Transformation:** The Wood Element embodies expansion, renewal, and personal evolution. Wood constitution individuals are often goal-oriented and deeply invested in self-improvement.

- **Purpose and Mission:** They often possess a deep connection to their life's purpose, inspired by justice, creativity, or a desire to bring new ideas into the world.

- **Bond with Nature:** Reflecting the qualities of trees and plants, Wood types people often feel extremely connected to the natural world, drawing vitality and inspiration from outdoor environments.

4. Maintaining Balance in the Wood Element

To maintain harmony within the Wood Element, it is essential to cultivate their physical, emotional, and spiritual well-being:

- **Physical Care:** Regular body movement, stretching, and flexibility exercises help to support the liver and gallbladder. Regular consumption of liver-friendly foods like leafy greens also promotes internal balance.

- **Emotional Regulation:** Journaling, meditation, mindfulness, and relaxation techniques can help process emotions and reduce stress. Cultivating adaptability and releasing rigid perfectionism contributes to emotional equilibrium.

- **Spiritual Nourishment:** Making time to be present in nature, engaging in continuous learning, and setting personal growth goals can cultivate a sense of fulfillment and alignment.

Constitution	Characteristics
Fire	Extrovert, easily excited, center of party, the "kisser," difficult to calm down-exaggerates, sharp mental activity
Earth	Honest, kind, maternal, laid back, easily satisfied, aloof from the world, slow to respond to stimulus
Metal	Broadminded, wise, rule follower, aloof, righteous, confident
Water	Introvert, quiet observer, fearful, deep thinker, can be fear biter, consistent but slow
Wood	Extrovert, dominant, impatient, vigilant, enjoys moving/running, quick tempered, changes mind easily

How Microtrauma Builds Strength

Our bodies are remarkably designed to respond, adapt, and grow stronger when exposed to controlled challenges. I have come to know of the body's natural response to minor injuries, as *The "Splinter Effect,"* (Birch, 2003; Birch and Felt, 1999). This term highlights the cascade of vascular and immune responses that occur after a puncture (such as from a splinter) or trauma, illustrating the body's ability to control damage, prevent infection, and facilitate tissue repair. This concept parallels established understandings of the inflammatory and healing processes, such as those detailed by Micozzi (2011).

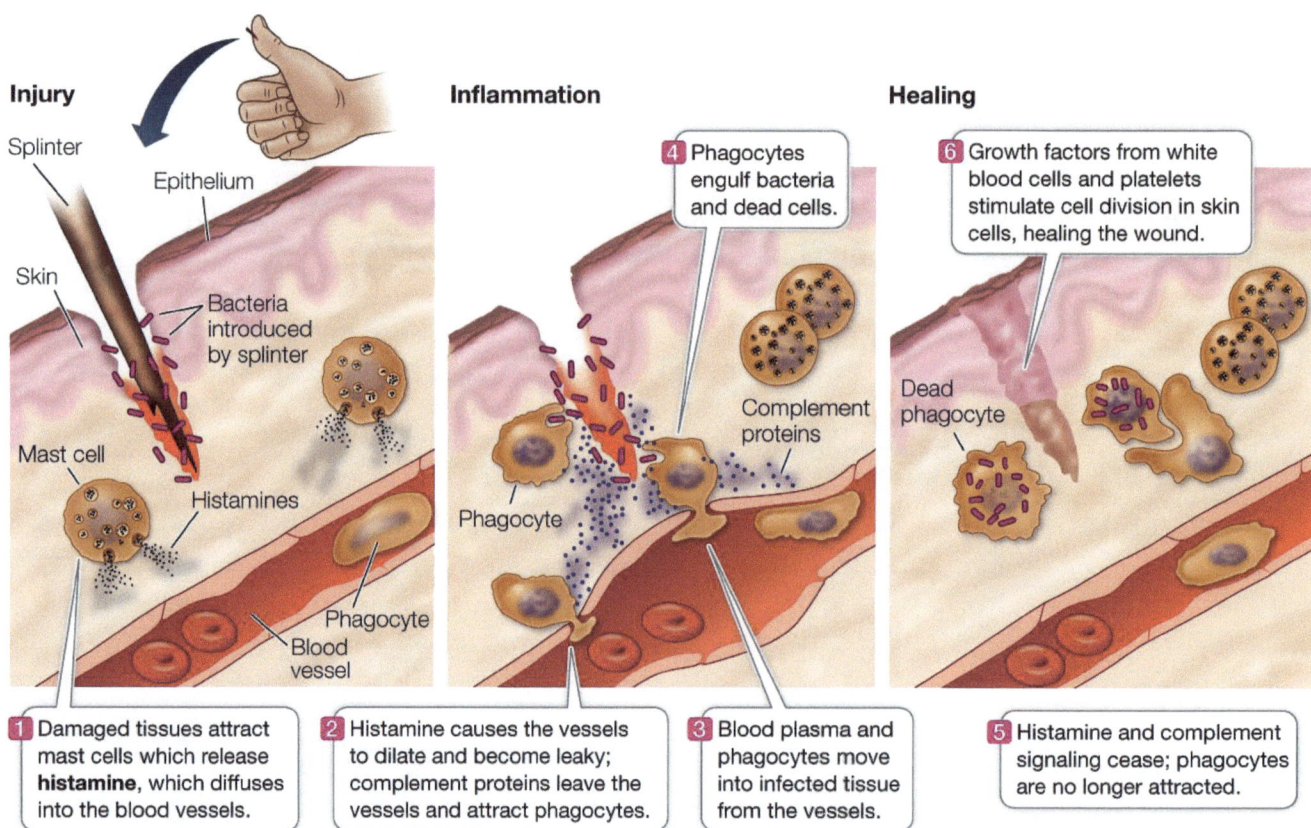

Injury — Splinter, Epithelium, Skin, Bacteria introduced by splinter, Mast cell, Histamines, Phagocyte, Blood vessel

Inflammation — 4 Phagocytes engulf bacteria and dead cells. Complement proteins, Phagocyte

Healing — 6 Growth factors from white blood cells and platelets stimulate cell division in skin cells, healing the wound. Dead phagocyte

1 Damaged tissues attract mast cells which release **histamine**, which diffuses into the blood vessels.

2 Histamine causes the vessels to dilate and become leaky; complement proteins leave the vessels and attract phagocytes.

3 Blood plasma and phagocytes move into infected tissue from the vessels.

5 Histamine and complement signaling cease; phagocytes are no longer attracted.

LIFE: THE SCIENCE OF BIOLOGY 11e, Figure 41.5
© 2017 Sinauer Associates, Inc.

Interestingly, this same biological principle applies to how the body responds to the small, intentional stresses placed on muscles, bones, and tissues through strategic physical exertion. This concept is also sometimes referred to as *exercise-induced microtrauma*, *strategic* or *hermetic trauma*. Just as the body heals and strengthens itself after encountering a splinter, it undergoes a similar process when recovering from the controlled damage caused by exercise, ultimately leading to increased strength, resilience, and adaptability.

Understanding the Splinter Effect

The Splinter Effect describes three distinct stages that occur in response to tissue damage:

1. Vasoconstriction: Immediate Defense (Duration: ~20 minutes)
- Blood vessels constrict to minimize blood loss and prevent the spread of microorganisms.

- The body contains the damage and initiates a defensive response.

2. Vasodilation: Recruitment of Immune Cells (Duration: 2 to 3 hours)
- Blood vessels widen to allow white blood cells and immune cells to reach the injured tissue.

- Increased circulation flushes out pathogens and initiates tissue repair.

3. Vasomotion: Microvascular Pumping (Duration: ~1 hour)
- Microscopic vessels oscillate to facilitate the removal of debris and damaged cells.

- Tissue is nourished, oxygenated, and prepared for repair and regeneration.

These vascular and metabolic changes ultimately promote healing and prepare the tissue for future challenges.

Exercise and the Microtrauma Connection: Building Strength Through Controlled Damage

When you engage in:

- resistance training
- high-intensity exercise
- strategic physical exertion

…you introduce a form of **microtrauma** to your muscles, tendons, and bones. While this might sound detrimental, this micro-damage is essential for adaptation and growth. The body responds to this stress by initiating a process remarkably similar to the Splinter Effect:

1. Vasoconstriction and Inflammatory Response (Initial 20-30 Minutes)
- Following intense exercise, tiny tears occur in muscle fibers, prompting an immediate vasoconstrictive response.

- Just like with a splinter, the body temporarily restricts blood flow to prevent excessive swelling and contain the initial damage.

2. Vasodilation and Immune Activation (2 to 3 Hours Post-Exercise)
- Shortly after the initial restriction, vasodilation occurs, allowing an influx of oxygen, nutrients, and immune cells to flood the damaged area.

- Macrophages and neutrophils break down damaged cells while stimulating the release of growth factors that promote tissue repair.

- This phase also enhances the removal of metabolic waste products like lactic acid, reducing post-exercise soreness.

3. Vasomotion and Tissue Remodeling (1 to 2 Hours After)
- During this phase, the rhythmic pulsing of micro vessels helps flush away damaged tissue and enhances the circulation of oxygen and nutrients.

- Fibroblasts and satellite cells initiate tissue repair, producing collagen and new muscle fibers to replace the damaged cells.

- This process strengthens the tissue, making it more resilient to future stress.

Bone Adaptation and Microtrauma: Building a Stronger Framework

Exercise not only strengthens muscles but also stimulates **bone remodeling** through a similar process. When bones experience microtrauma from weight-bearing or high-impact activities:

- **Osteoblasts** are activated to deposit new bone tissue.

- Over time, bones become denser and stronger in response to increased mechanical stress.

- This mechanism helps prevent osteoporosis and enhances bone resilience, especially when combined with adequate nutrition, including vitamin D and calcium.

The bone remodeling process

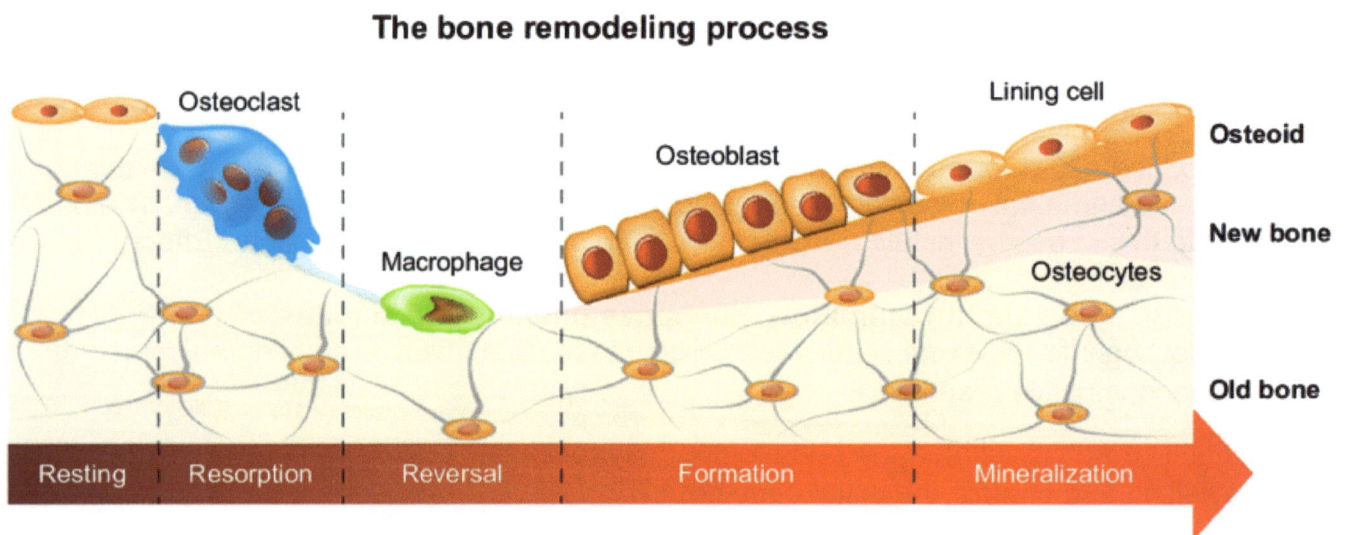

Bone Remodeling

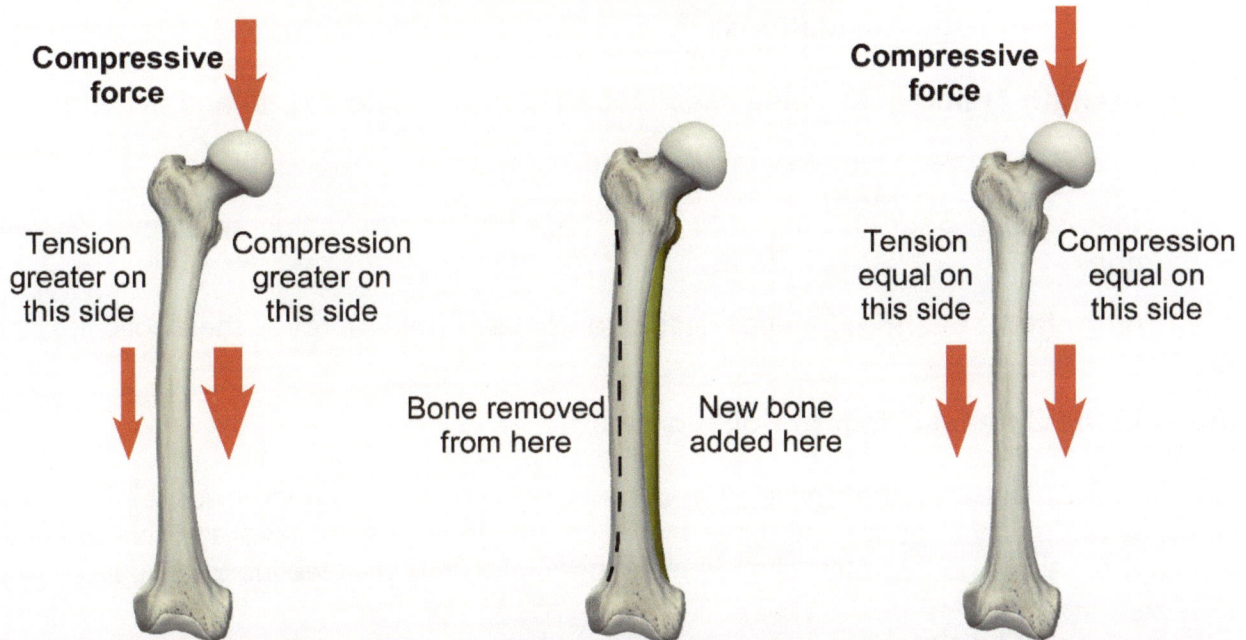

Compressive force

Tension greater on this side | Compression greater on this side

Compressive force

Tension equal on this side | Compression equal on this side

Bone removed from here | New bone added here

The application of force to a slightly bent bone produces a greater compressive force on the inside curvature. compressive force produces weak electrical currents (action potentials) which stimulate osteoblast production.

Over time, bone matrix is deposited on the inside curvature and removed from the outside curvature.

The final result is a bone matched to the compressive force to which it is exposed.

www.MindandBodyExercises.com

© Copyright 2021 - CAD Graphics, Inc.

The Role of Strategic Trauma in Cardiovascular Adaptation

Interestingly, the cardiovascular system also benefits from controlled stress. Aerobic and high-intensity interval training (HIIT) create microtrauma and oxidative stress within the vascular system:

- Endothelial cells release **nitric oxide**, promoting vasodilation and improving blood vessel flexibility.

- Over time, regular cardiovascular stress leads to the growth of new capillaries, enhancing circulation and oxygen delivery to tissues.

The Principle of Hormesis: What Doesn't Kill You Makes You Stronger

The biological response to controlled microtrauma is an example of *hormesis*, a process where exposure to mild stress stimulates adaptive responses that make the body stronger.

Just as repeated exposure to small challenges prepares the body for more significant threats, strategic trauma through exercise enhances strength, resilience, and longevity.

Examples of Hermetic Adaptations:

- **Strength Training:** Microtears in muscle fibers stimulate growth and hypertrophy.

- **Cold Exposure:** Promotes vasoconstriction and metabolic adaptation.

- **Heat Stress (Sauna):** Enhances heat shock protein production and improves cellular repair.

- **Intermittent Fasting:** Induces cellular autophagy and improves metabolic flexibility.

Applying the Splinter Effect to Holistic Health

The correlation between the *Splinter Effect* and exercise-induced microtrauma highlights the body's innate ability to adapt and thrive under controlled stress. To leverage this adaptive capacity, consider incorporating the following principles into your wellness routine:

1. Progressive Overload
Gradually increase the intensity, duration, or resistance of your exercise routine to continually challenge your body and promote adaptation.

2. Adequate Recovery
Just as the body needs time to repair after a splinter wound, adequate rest and recovery are essential for tissue repair and growth following intense exercise.

3. Anti-Inflammatory Nutrition
Support tissue healing by consuming anti-inflammatory foods rich in antioxidants, omega-3 fatty acids, and essential vitamins and minerals.

4. Mindful Stress Management
Manage external stressors to ensure that the body's adaptive responses are not overwhelmed by chronic inflammation, which can inhibit proper healing and adaptation.

Conclusion: Strength Through Controlled Challenge

The Splinter Effect beautifully illustrates how the body responds to injury by initiating a cascade of vascular and immune responses that promote healing and strengthen tissues. This same biological mechanism underlies how strategic trauma through exercise and controlled stress transforms the body, enhancing strength, endurance, and resilience. By understanding and embracing these natural processes, we can optimize our fitness, protect against injury, and cultivate a body that thrives under pressure, just as nature intended.

References:

Birch S, Felt R. (1999) Understanding acupuncture. Churchill Livingstone: London
Micozzi, Marc S. (2011) Fundamentals of Complementary, Alternative, and Integrative
Medicine - E-Book (p. 536). Elsevier Health Sciences. Kindle Edition
.
Peake, J., Neubauer, O., Della Gatta, P., & Nosaka, K. (2017). Muscle damage and
inflammation during recovery from exercise. *Journal of Applied Physiology, 122*(3), 559-570.
https://doi.org/10.1152/japplphysiol.00971.2016

Schoenfeld, B. J. (2010). The mechanisms of muscle hypertrophy and their application to
resistance training. *Journal of Strength and Conditioning Research, 24*(10), 2857-2872.
https://doi.org/10.1519/JSC.0b013e3181e840f3

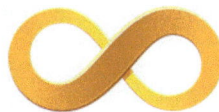

Are Food Preservatives "Preserving" Health Risks in the Body?

The potential for preservatives and other food additives to have long-term effects on human health has indeed been a subject of research and debate. While the preservatives used in food are generally approved by regulatory agencies and deemed safe within established limits, or "generally recognized as safe" (GRAS), there is concern about how these substances might interact with the human body, particularly with prolonged exposure or high consumption levels.

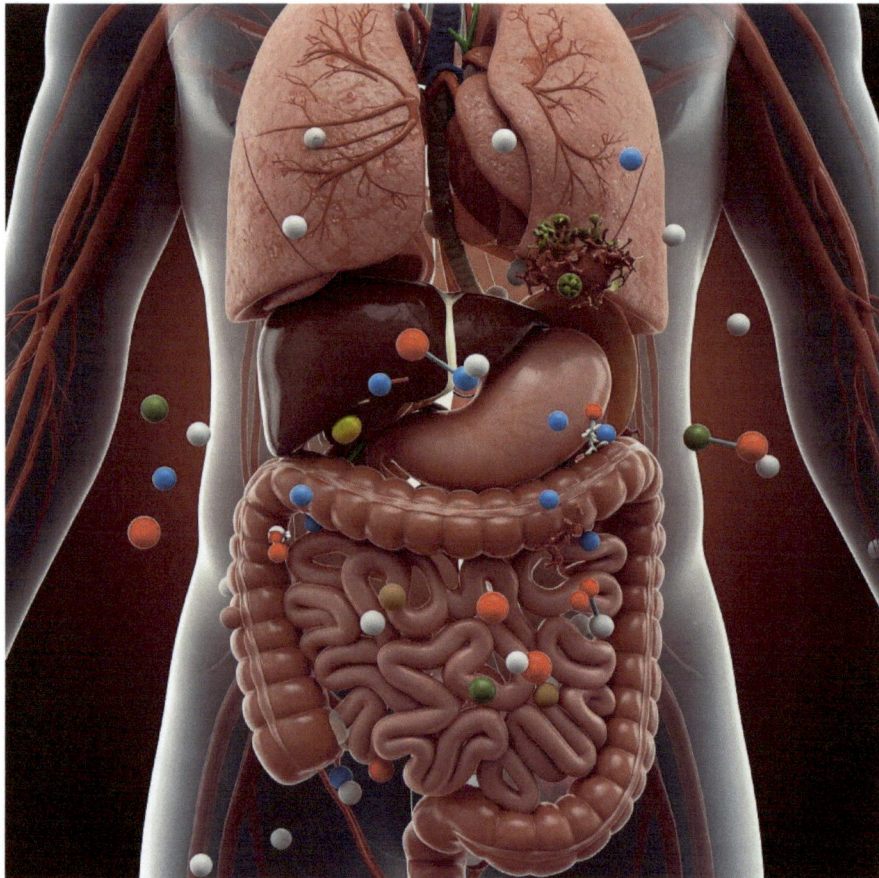

Many preservatives target microbial cells rather than human cells, and they often break down or are excreted from the body. However, some studies suggest certain preservatives might contribute to adverse health effects, such as inflammation, gut microbiome disruption, or oxidative stress (Zhou et al., 2023).

Some examples:

- **Sodium benzoate** is widely used in acidic foods like sodas and fruit juices. Research has shown that under certain conditions, it can convert to benzene, a known carcinogen, especially when combined with ascorbic acid (vitamin C) (McNeal et al., 1993). The risk is generally low, but it raises concerns about high levels of consumption.

- **Nitrates and nitrites**, commonly found in processed meats, can convert into nitrosamines in the stomach, compounds associated with an increased risk of cancers such as colorectal cancer (Song et al., 2015).

- **BHT and BHA** are synthetic antioxidants used in fats and oils to prevent rancidity. There is some evidence that they may act as endocrine disruptors and impact cellular processes, although results are mixed (Pop et al., 2013).

The body's detoxification systems, primarily the liver and kidneys, are generally effective at processing and eliminating many of these compounds. However, researchers argue that cumulative effects from chronic exposure to multiple food additives, combined with other dietary and lifestyle factors, could potentially pose health risks over time (Witkowska et al., 2021). We have known for many decades that a balanced diet with minimally processed foods can help to reduce exposure to these additives, though experts always state that more research is needed to understand their long-term impacts fully. The FDA finally banned red dye in the U.S. for use in cosmetics back in 1990 but not in foods until just January of 2025 (Davis, 2025).

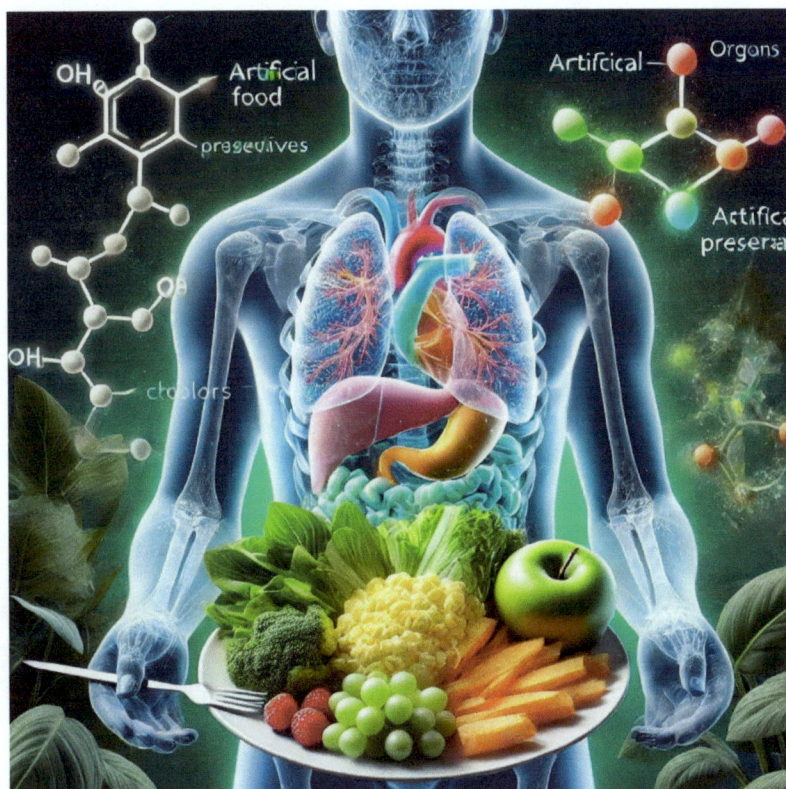

References:

Zhou, X., Qiao, K., Wu, H., & Zhang, Y. (2023). The Impact of Food Additives on the Abundance and Composition of Gut Microbiota. Molecules (Basel, Switzerland), 28(2), 631. https://doi.org/10.3390/molecules28020631

McNeal, T. P., Nyman, P. J., Benson, J. M., & Diachenko, G. W. (1993). Survey of benzene in foods by using headspace concentration techniques and capillary gas chromatography. Journal of AOAC International, 76(6), 1213-1219.

Song, P., Wu, L., & Guan, W. (2015). Dietary Nitrates, Nitrites, and Nitrosamines Intake and the Risk of Gastric Cancer: A Meta-Analysis. Nutrients, 7(12), 9872–9895. https://doi.org/10.3390/nu7125505

Pop, A., Kiss, B., & Loghin, F. (2013). Endocrine disrupting effects of butylated hydroxyanisole (BHA – E320). Clujul medical (1957), 86(1), 16–20.

Witkowska, D., Słowik, J., & Chilicka, K. (2021). Heavy Metals and Human Health: Possible Exposure Pathways and the Competition for Protein Binding Sites. Molecules (Basel, Switzerland), 26(19), 6060. https://doi.org/10.3390/molecules26196060

Davis, Josh, How Red Dye 3 finally got banned in foods, according to a dietitian. (2025). https://www.houstonmethodist.org/blog/articles/2024/may/is-red-dye-no-3-in-food-bad-for-you-a-dieticians-take/

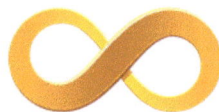

SECTION III: Movement Practices for Health

Yoga Is More Than Glorified Stretching

As a practitioner of martial arts (kung fu and styles of Tai Chi and BaguaZhang), yoga, qigong, and dao yin (martial arts yoga) for over 40 years, I can vouch for the vast amount of mental and physical benefits that not only have I received, but others that I have either taught or trained with. Qigong and martial arts are deeply rooted in the 8 Limbs of Ayurveda, and concerning this post, yogic practices of asanas or physical postures.

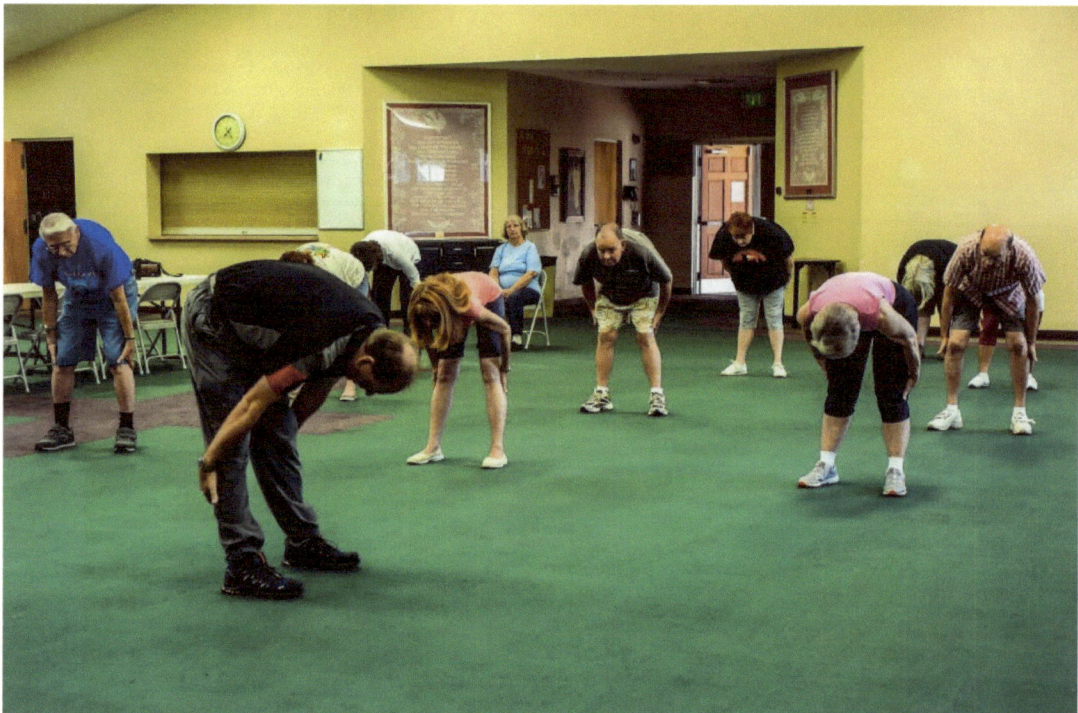

The BBC article "How Yoga Can Rewire Your Brain and Improve Your Mental Health" discusses recent findings on how yoga practice can have effects on brain structure and function, highlighting its potential mental health benefits. Recent research indicates that regular yoga practice can lead to physical changes in the brain, such as increased gray matter, which is associated with improved cognitive functions and emotional regulation. These neurological alterations may contribute to symptoms of less anxiety and depression. The article emphasizes that yoga's combination of physical postures, breathing exercises, and meditation not only enhances physical well-being but also offers significant mental health advantages. For the purpose of my post, I will refer to yoga, qigong, and dao yin interchangeably, as they all are on some level the same type of physical, mental, and spiritual exercises.

The Science Behind Yoga (Qigong & Dao Yin): How It Rewires Your Brain and Enhances Mental Health

In recent years, yoga has gained more widespread recognition not just for its physical benefits but also for its significant impact on mental well-being. Research now suggests that regular and consistent yoga practice can help to rewire the brain, improving cognitive function, emotional regulation, and stress management. How do these ancient practices impact modern neuroscience? I will summarize some amazing connections between these mind-body practices and brain health.

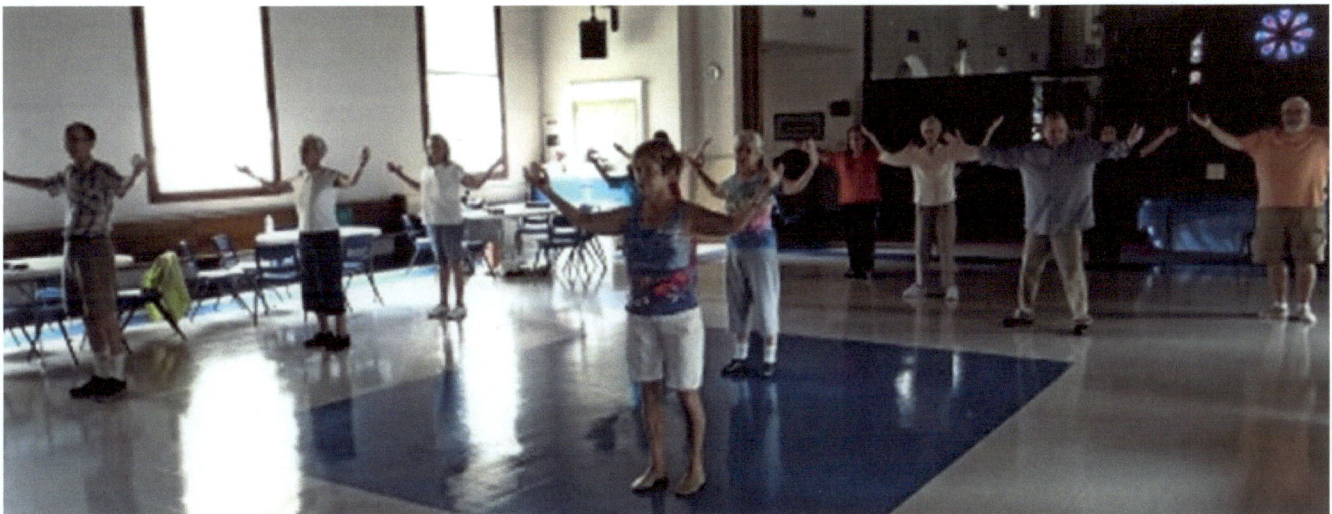

How Yoga Affects the Brain

Enhancing Neuroplasticity

Yoga has been shown to promote neuroplasticity, which is the brain's ability to reorganize and form new neural connections. Research studies using MRI scans have found increased gray matter density in the hippocampus and prefrontal cortex of yoga practitioners. These areas are important for memory, self-awareness, and emotional regulation, suggesting that yoga can help individuals become more adaptable to stress and improve various cognitive functions.

Neuroplasticity

Dancing, yoga, tai chi and other mind and body practices increases neural connectivity.

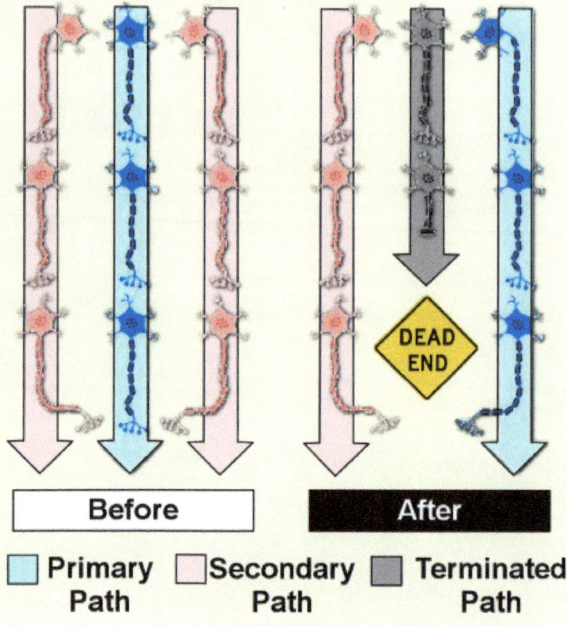

Rerouting: New neural connections are made between active neurons to create alternate neural pathways.

Before
After
DEAD END

Primary Path
Secondary Path
Terminated Path

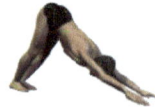
Yoga

Tai Chi

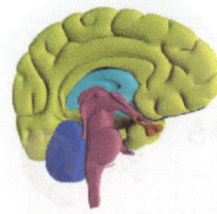

Meditation

Baguazhang

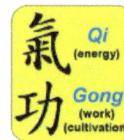
氣功 *Qi* (energy) *Gong* (work) (cultivation)

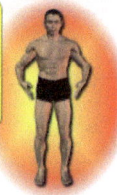

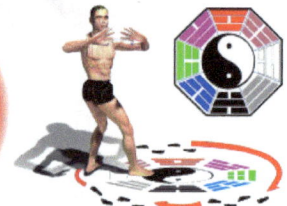

www.MindAndBodyExercises.com

Reducing Anxiety and Depression

One of yoga's most significant mental health benefits is its ability to alleviate anxiety and depression. Research indicates that yoga decreases cortisol, the body's primary stress hormone, while boosting gamma-aminobutyric acid (GABA), a neurotransmitter that promotes relaxation. These biochemical changes contribute to a calmer, more balanced state of mind, making yoga an effective tool for managing mood disorders.

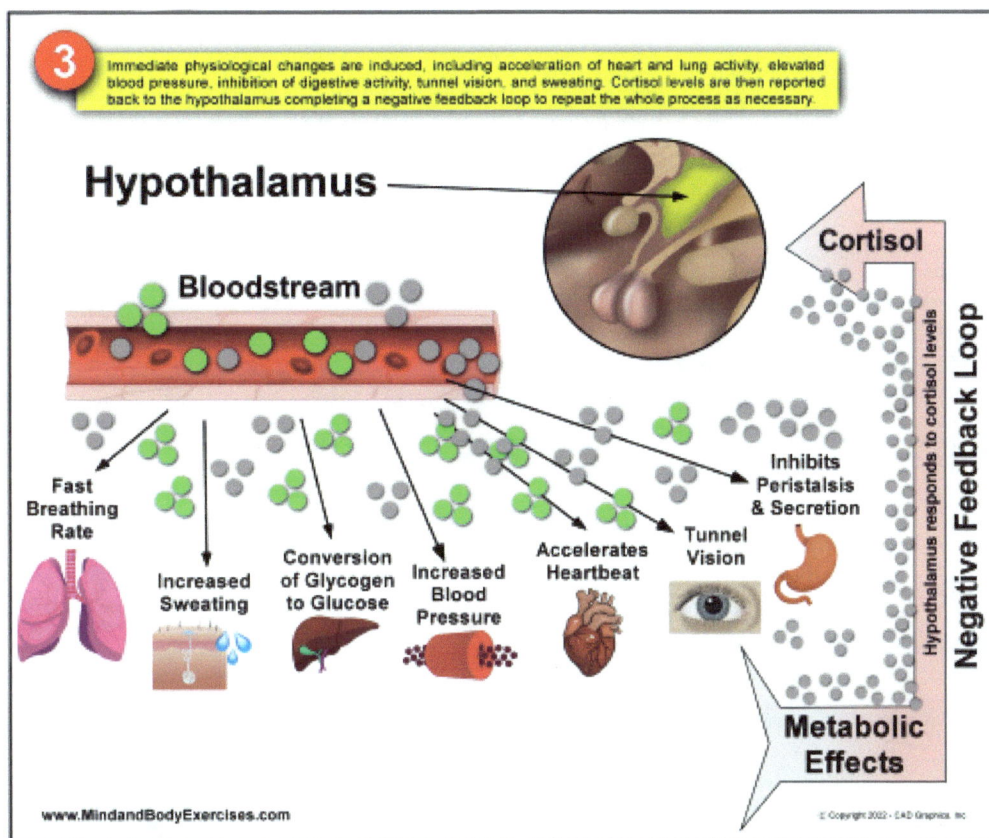

3 Immediate physiological changes are induced, including acceleration of heart and lung activity, elevated blood pressure, inhibition of digestive activity, tunnel vision, and sweating. Cortisol levels are then reported back to the hypothalamus completing a negative feedback loop to repeat the whole process as necessary.

Hypothalamus

Bloodstream

Cortisol

Fast Breathing Rate

Increased Sweating

Conversion of Glycogen to Liver

Increased Blood Pressure

Accelerates Heartbeat

Tunnel Vision

Inhibits Peristalsis & Secretion

Hypothalamus responds to cortisol levels

Negative Feedback Loop

Metabolic Effects

www.MindandBodyExercises.com

© Copyright 2022 - CAD Graphics, Inc

The Role of Breathwork and Meditation

Beyond the asanas or physical postures, yoga incorporates breathwork (pranayama) and meditation, both of which play a vital role in mental health. Deep, regulated breathing stimulates the parasympathetic nervous system, reducing the body's fight-or-flight response. Meditation fosters mindfulness, promoting present-moment awareness and reduction of rumination, two key factors in maintaining emotional stability.

Cognitive Benefits and Emotional Regulation

Practicing yoga and other mind-body methods have been linked to increased cognitive function, including better focus, memory, and decision-making. The increased activity in the prefrontal cortex enhances executive functions, allowing individuals to better manage stress more effectively and respond to challenges with greater clarity.

Yoga as a Holistic Mental Health Solution

Pharmaceutical treatments usually target specific symptoms, whereas yoga offers a comprehensive approach to mental wellness. By integrating physical movement, breath control, and mindfulness, yoga cultivates overall brain health and emotional resilience. Whether practicing at a studio, school, outdoors, or at home, yoga, qigong, and dao yin provide a natural, often inexpensive, and accessible way to improve mental well-being.

Final Thoughts

To me, the evidence is quite clear that the mind-body methods of yoga, qigong, and daoyin are not just a workout; they are powerful tools for brain health and mental clarity. By supplementing some of these methods into your routine, you can strengthen your mind, reduce stress, and cultivate emotional balance. Whether you're a beginner or an experienced practitioner, the benefits of these extend far beyond the mat or studio, offering a holistic path to overall well-being.

Tai chi, one of the most well-known Chinese martial arts, has evolved significantly as it has spread beyond China. Originally developed as an internal martial art (*neijia*) integrating martial applications, health benefits, and Daoist philosophical principles, tai chi has often been misrepresented in the United States. While many instructors have contributed positively to promoting its health benefits, others have mischaracterized the art, not necessarily by teaching bad practices, but by presenting something entirely different under the tai chi name. Having practiced, studied, and researched martial arts for over 40 years, and legitimate tai chi for the last 25 years, I have personally witnessed the bait-and-switch tactics used to market tai chi to Western audiences. Some instructors, either due to a lack of proper training or deliberate deception, have claimed to teach authentic tai chi while actually presenting simplified qigong exercises, unrelated movement drills, or incomplete systems. While qigong and tai chi are both respected Chinese internal arts, they are not interchangeable. All tai chi is qigong, but not all qigong is tai chi. This misrepresentation undermines the integrity of an institution built on discipline, honesty, and tradition.

This article examines the philosophical foundations of tai chi, its key physical components, and the ways to identify authentic practice, particularly within the *Chen*, *Yang*, and *Wu* styles, which are three prominent traditional lineages.

Firsthand Observations of Tai Chi's Migration and "Bait-and-Switch"

When tai chi was first introduced in the United States, several Asian martial artists took advantage of the limited understanding of internal martial arts among Western practitioners. Some presented adjusted qigong sequences or simplified slow-motion movements as "tai chi," presuming that American students would not discern the difference.

A fitting analogy for this phenomenon can be seen in the restaurant industry. Imagine going to a Chinese restaurant and ordering the Korean dish *"bi bim bop."* The menu lists it clearly, so you expect to receive the correct dish. But when the server brings your meal, you are given *"lo mein"* noodles instead, and they insist that this is bi bim bop. While lo mein is still an Asian dish, and perhaps even delicious, it is NOT what you ordered.

This is exactly what has happened with tai chi in the West. Many students sign up for classes expecting to learn a legitimate tai chi lineage, yet what they receive is a completely different system, usually a generic set of slow movements, breathwork, or unrelated qigong exercises.

Another analogy would be a student enrolling in a college program to earn a degree in Cantonese. They spend four years diligently studying, assuming they are learning the language they signed up for. However, upon graduation, they realize they have actually been taught Mandarin instead. While Mandarin is still a valuable language, the fact remains that the institution misled the student about what they were learning.

Starting.	Parting The Wild Horse's Mane. 3 times.	White Crane Spreads It's Wings.	Brush Knee, Push. 3 times.	Playing The Guitar/Lute/Pipa.	Repulse Monkey. 4 times.	Hold The Ball, Ward Off.
Grasp The Bird's Tail.	Press, Sit Back.	Open up and Push. Repeat the last 4 moves, going right.	Single Whip.	Cloud Hands, going left.	Single Whip again, High Pat on Horse.	Right Heel Kick.
Carry The Tiger Over The Mountain.	Turn.	Left Heel Kick.	Snake Creeps Through The Grass.	Stand on one leg. Repeat on Right side.	Shuttle Back And Forth.	Needle At Bottom Of The Sea.
Fan Through The Back.	Turn.	Right Back Fist.	Parry and Punch.	Apparent Closing.	Cross Hands.	Close.

This **IS** Tai Chi, Yang 24 with names for each exercise

Similarly, in the world of tai chi, many instructors have claimed to teach legitimate Chen, Yang, or Wu styles tai chi, but in reality, what they teach lacks core structural components, martial applications, key internal mechanics and philosophy of these arts as a whole. While what they offer may still provide health benefits, students deserve transparency about what they are actually learning.

I have personally encountered numerous instructors who claimed to teach authentic tai chi but omitted core elements such as silk-reeling energy (*Chan Si Jin*), *fajin* (explosive power), and martial applications. Similarly, other teachers abandoned tai chi's rooting, structural integrity, and push hands training, reducing the practice to mere choreographed relaxation exercises or maybe physical fitness methods at best.

This misrepresentation, while sometimes unintentional and others deliberately misleading, is problematic because martial arts in general and tai chi in particular, are institutions that pride themselves on high moral standards, integrity, and character. The issue is not that what these instructors teach is inherently bad or ineffective. Many of these adapted forms still provide great health and self-defense benefits. However, they have misrepresented their systems as part of a legitimate lineage when they are not.

With greater access to legitimate sources, historical records, and international training opportunities, modern practitioners can now recognize the discrepancies between traditional tai chi and commercialized adaptations. However, the impact of this bait-and-switch phenomenon still lingers in the tai chi landscape today.

Philosophical Foundations of Tai Chi

Tai chi is deeply rooted in Daoist and Confucian philosophy, *incorporating yin-yang theory*, Five Element Theory (*Wu Xing*), and *Bagua* (Eight Trigrams theory). These principles shape both physical movements and the strategic martial applications of the art.

The Five Aspects of Yin and Yang

The 5 Aspects of yin and yang complement and balance each other via these aspects, which define the relationship between each.

1) Opposition

2) Interdependence

3) Mutual Consuming-Increasing

4) Mutual Transforming

5) Infinite Divisibility

www.MindAndBodyExercises.com   © Copyright 2024 - CAD Graphics, Inc.

Yin and Yang: The Balance of Softness and Strength

Tai chi, literally translated as "Supreme Ultimate", embodies the interplay of yin (softness, receptivity) and yang (hardness, action). Movements transition fluidly between yielding and attacking, expansion and contraction, in accordance with these principles.

This balance is evident across all major styles:

- *Chen*-style integrates sudden explosive releases of energy (*fajin*) alongside soft, coiling movements.

- *Yang*-style, derived from Chen, smooths out the transitions but retains the root structure and internal power.

- *Wu*-style, known for its compact, small-frame movements, emphasizes yielding and subtle redirections over forceful exchanges.

The Five Elements (Wu Xing) in Tai Chi Practice

The Five Element Theory (Wu Xing) describes dynamic interactions in nature, which tai chi integrates into its movement and energy principles. Each element correlates with essential aspects of tai chi's execution:

- **Wood (expansion, spiraling energy)** – Silk-reeling movements (Chen-style) and the extension of intent through structure (Yang & Wu styles).

- **Fire (ascending, explosive power)** – Fajin (Chen-style), as well as the expansive issuing energy in Yang and Wu applications.

- **Earth (stability, neutrality)** – Rooting and central equilibrium across all tai chi styles.

- **Metal (condensing, refining force)** – The precision of structure and economy of movement, particularly in Wu-style's compact footwork.

- **Water (flow, adaptability)** – The continuous, uninterrupted movement quality of Yang and Wu styles, contrasted with the coiling, wave-like motions of Chen-style.

The 5 Root Powers of Tai Chi

The fundamental practices of Tai Chi are based upon 13 postures. These 13 postures consist of 8 forces, or "expressions of energy", and 5 steps, root powers or directions of movement.

Tui Wood (back)

5 Elements - Wu Xing

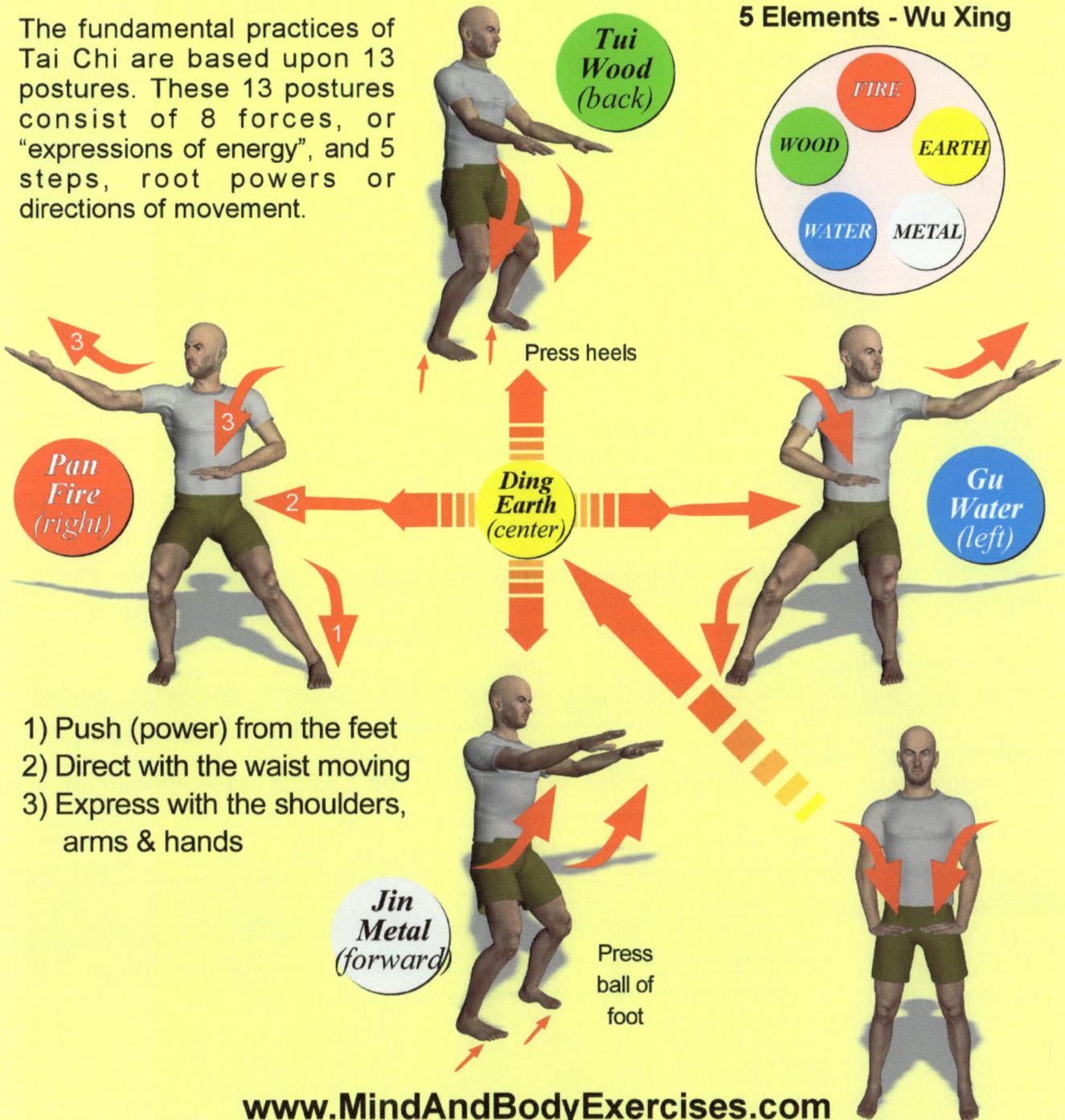

FIRE

WOOD

EARTH

WATER

METAL

Press heels

Ding Earth (center)

Pan Fire (right)

Gu Water (left)

1) Push (power) from the feet
2) Direct with the waist moving
3) Express with the shoulders, arms & hands

Jin Metal (forward)

Press ball of foot

www.MindAndBodyExercises.com

© Copyright 2020 - CAD Graphics, Inc.

Bagua (Eight Trigrams) and Cycles of Transformation

Tai chi shares conceptual similarities with Bagua Zhang (Eight Trigrams Palm), particularly in its circular stepping and understanding of transformation in combat. The eight trigrams (Bagua) symbolize natural forces of heaven, earth, wind, thunder, water, fire, mountain, and valley where each influence different movement qualities.

The 8 energies of fundamental tai chi principles correspond with the 8 trigrams of the bagua:

- **Peng (heaven) - Ward Off:**
This energy is about expanding outwards and destabilizing an opponent, likened to a filling balloon.

- **Lu (earth) - Roll Back:**
This energy involves a rolling or drawing action while grounding and stabilizing, like drawing a line with a brush.

- **Ji (water) - Press:**
This energy involves a squeezing or pressing action, often used to control an opponent's movement.

- **An (fire) - Push:**
This energy is a direct pushing action, used to move an opponent away or to create an opening.

- **Tsai (wind) - Pluck:**
This energy is a plucking, pulling or grabbing action, used to disrupt an opponent's balance.

- **Lieh (thunder) - Split:**
This energy involves a splitting or parting action, used to create space or to separate an opponent.

- **Zhou (valley) - Elbow:** This energy uses the elbow as a weapon, either for striking or for blocking.

- **Kao (mountain) - Shoulder:** This energy uses the shoulder to bump or lean into an opponent, creating an opportunity for attack or defense.

The 8 Expressions, 8 Energies, 8 Principles of Tai Chi

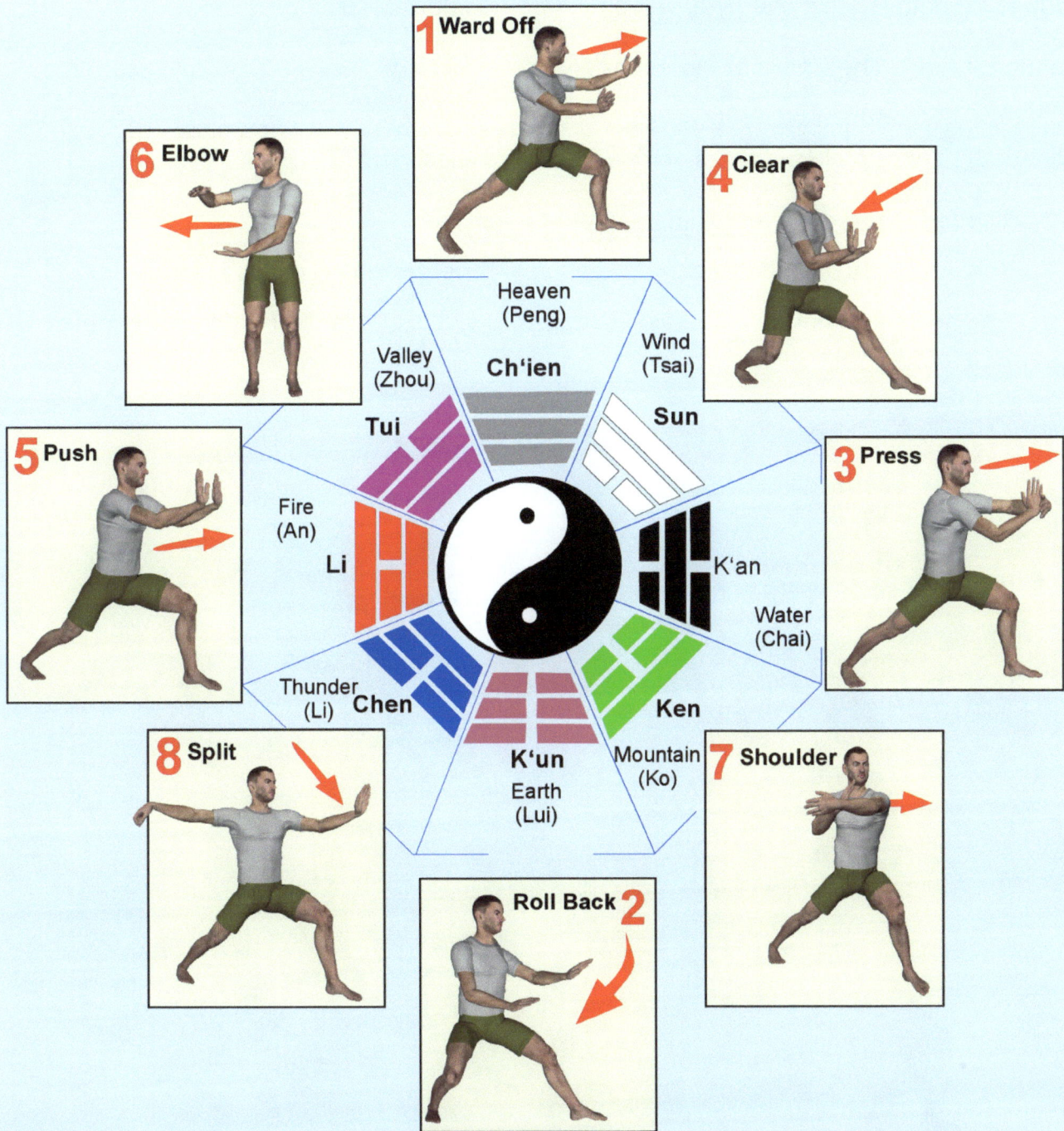

1 Ward Off

4 Clear

6 Elbow

5 Push

8 Split

3 Press

7 Shoulder

Roll Back 2

Heaven (Peng)

Valley (Zhou)

Wind (Tsai)

Ch'ien

Sun

Tui

Fire (An)

Li

K'an

Water (Chai)

Thunder (Li) **Chen**

Ken

K'un

Earth (Lui)

Mountain (Ko)

www.MindAndBodyExercises.com

© Copyright 2020 - CAD Graphics, Inc.

Physical Components of Authentic Tai Chi

Having personally trained with high-level practitioners from traditional tai chi lineages; I can confirm that authentic practice requires adherence to specific biomechanical principles. Many modern adaptations focus solely on relaxation, neglecting the essential physical structure required for both internal energy development and combat application.

Kinetic Linking: The Chain of Movement

Tai chi follows the principle of kinetic linking, where movement flows seamlessly through the entire body. This structure applies across all major styles:

1. **The feet root** – Power originates from the ground.

2. **The waist and spine direct** – The *dantian* (energy center) leads all movement.

3. **The arms and hands express** – Energy manifests outward through an integrated whole-body structure.

Feet - Waist - Arms - Kinetic Linking www.MindandBodyExercises.com

The Relationship Between a Tree and the Human Body

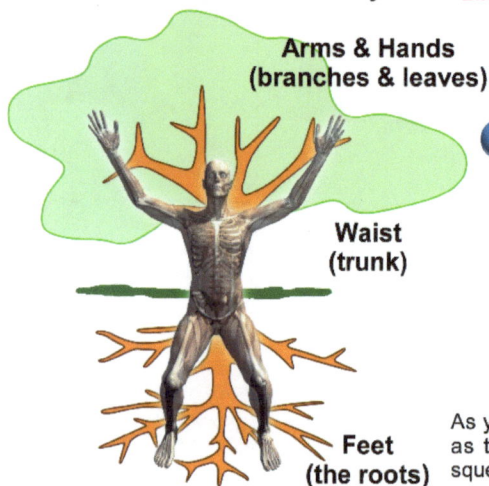

Kinetic - pertaining to movement or motion

Linking - to connect, unite

Arms & Hands (branches & leaves)

Waist (trunk)

Feet (the roots)

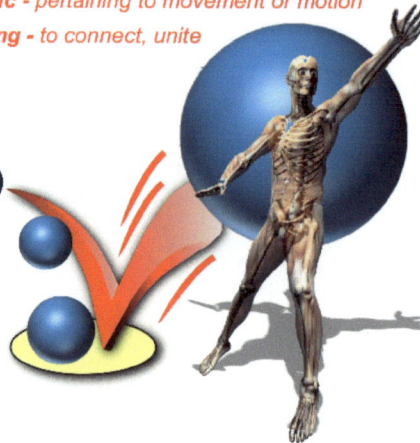

Many martial artists have known for maybe hundreds of years, that kinetic linking is a key factor in developing power for self defense skills as well as a way of improving overall fitness.

As you shift the weight from the back foot to the front foot, the waist, turns as the back extends forward and the arm reaches outward. Similar to squeezing a tube of toothpaste, from one end to the opposite, this motion consequently drives the force (along with blood and lymph) through the joints and blood vessels of the body in a flowing, fluid and spiralling motion.

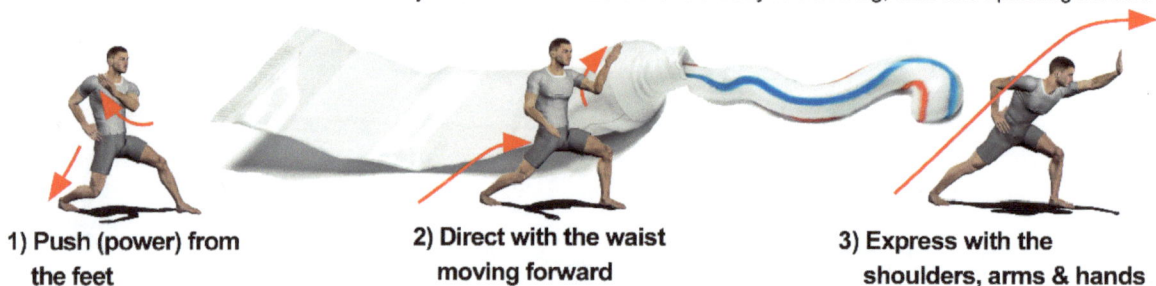

1) Push (power) from the feet

2) Direct with the waist moving forward

3) Express with the shoulders, arms & hands

Recognizing Authentic Chen, Yang, and Wu Tai Chi

Chen-Style Tai Chi
- **Alternating slow and fast movements** – Not just slow-motion practice.

- **Silk-reeling drills** – Without these, it is not real Chen-style tai chi.

- **Explosive fajin strikes** – Demonstrating internal power expression.

Yang-Style Tai Chi
- **Large, flowing postures** – Emphasis on balance and smoothness.

- **No abrupt power releases** – Unlike Chen-style, Yang-style minimizes fajin.

Wu-Style Tai Chi
- **Smaller movements and compact footwork** – Close-range efficiency.

- **Subtle redirections** – Making use of yielding and sensitivity.

Conclusion

As someone who has spent over four decades practicing, studying, and researching tai chi and other martial arts, I have personally witnessed both authentic and misrepresented versions of tai chi in the United States. While many well-intentioned teachers have promoted tai chi's health benefits, others have knowingly or unknowingly diluted the art, leading to confusion among students seeking traditional training. If a martial arts master, expert, instructor, etc., is going to invest their time, effort, and passion in teaching others, why not just spend the time and learn one of the original legitimate styles? Perhaps it is easier for them to keep perpetuating the deception, rather than learn the authentic styles? An elevated ego maybe, where one cannot accept that they have more to learn?

The bait-and-switch marketing model has been a persistent issue, with many instructors selling qigong exercises such as tai chi, stripping the art of its core biomechanical principles and martial applications. However, today's practitioners have more access to knowledge than ever before. By asking the right questions, studying traditional principles, and seeking qualified lineage-based instruction, students can ensure they are learning true, authentic tai chi, rather than an imitation product rebranded for unknowing students and even health care professionals that associate with these practices.

This issue extends beyond martial arts circles. Healthcare professionals, wellness coaches, and others who incorporate tai chi into their practices should be held to a higher standard of ethical responsibility. Professions that pride themselves on education and evidence-based care must ensure that what they promote aligns with authentic traditions, not diluted versions repackaged for commercial appeal. By failing to verify authenticity, they risk misleading their patients and clients, ultimately undermining trust and diminishing the effectiveness of these ancient practices. In a world where information is readily available, there is little excuse for perpetuating misconceptions. Upholding the integrity of both martial arts and healthcare professions requires a commitment to truth, accountability, and respect for the original systems that have endured for centuries.

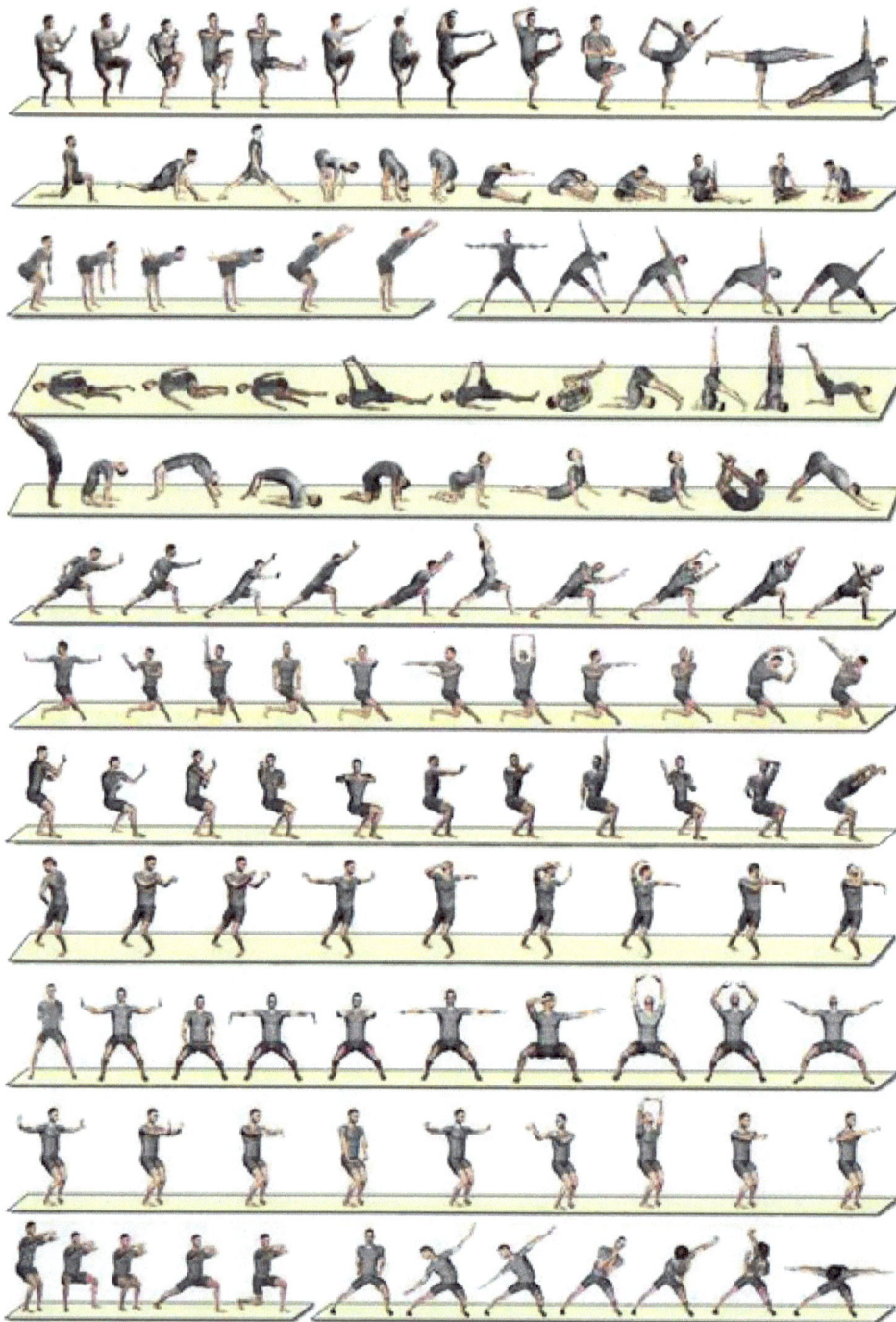

Daoist Yoga - DaoYi - Hard Qigong www.MindAndBody Exercises.com

*This **IS NOT** Tai Chi, but rather qigong or dao yin*

78

Fascia and Energy Flow

Unlocking the Link Between Myofascial Trains and TCM Meridians

Recent research has found links in form and function between the interactions of the fascial network and acupuncture. Health and fitness researchers have discovered that connective tissue, along with collagen fibers and fibroblasts, wraps around the end of the acupuncture needle when it is rotated in place. These effects have been seen at up to 4cm away from the site of needle insertion. Researchers have surmised that acupuncture energy meridians may follow the intermuscular or intramuscular myofascial lines. The myofascial meridians do not follow the precise lines of the Chinese energy meridians, which are an energetic connection rather than physical. However, there is some definite overlap. The unrestricted movement, taught in the Chinese internal martial arts, involves the free flow of Qi and aligning the myofascial lines (Yunshan et al., 2025).

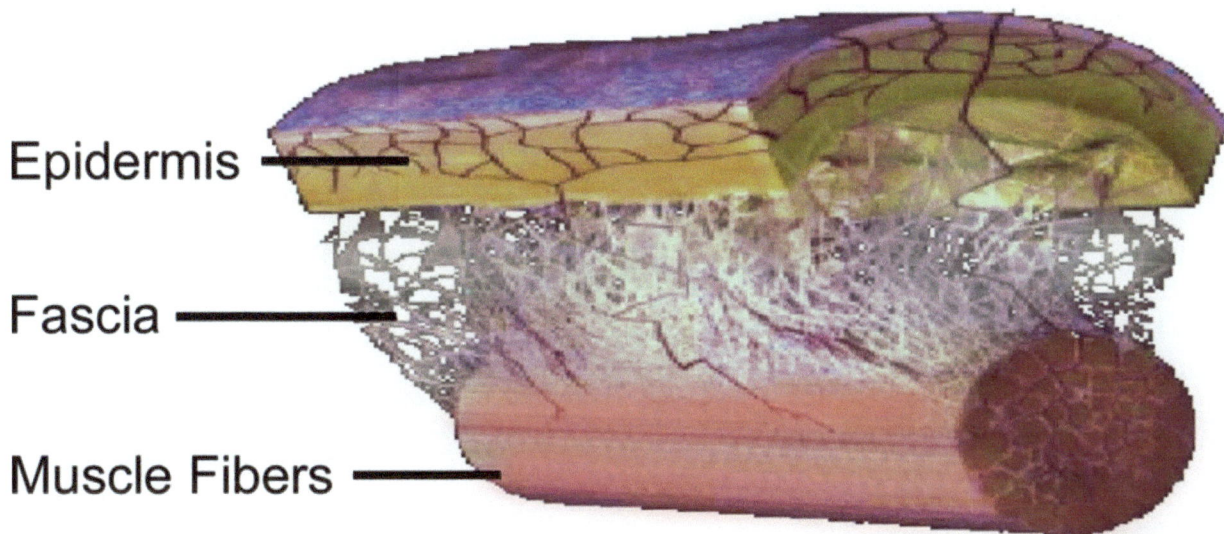

The connection between Traditional Chinese Medicine (TCM) meridians and the myofascial trains described in modern anatomy, particularly by Thomas Myers in *Anatomy Trains*, is a fascinating area of study. This relationship bridges ancient wisdom with contemporary science, offering insights into how energy and structure interact within the human body.

An Acupuncture Mechanism Theory

1 Pain manifests where a fascial triad (veins, arteries and nerves) is choked by collagen.

2 Free endings of veins, arteries and nerves (fascial triad) are roughly 82% identical to the 361 acupoints on the human body.

3 Needle is inserted at acupoints and then manipulated by twisting the needle thereby deforming the collagen of the fascia.

4 Choked collagen is deformed by the acupuncture needle, causing piezoelectric forces or pressure signals to be relayed via neural network.

interneuron pathways to the brain

dorsal root ganglion

spinal cord

Acupuncture Needle

Epidermis

Dermis

0.5-4mm thick

Hypodermis

Fascia

Muscle

© Copyright 2021 - CAD Graphics, Inc.

The 12 Primary Energy Meridians

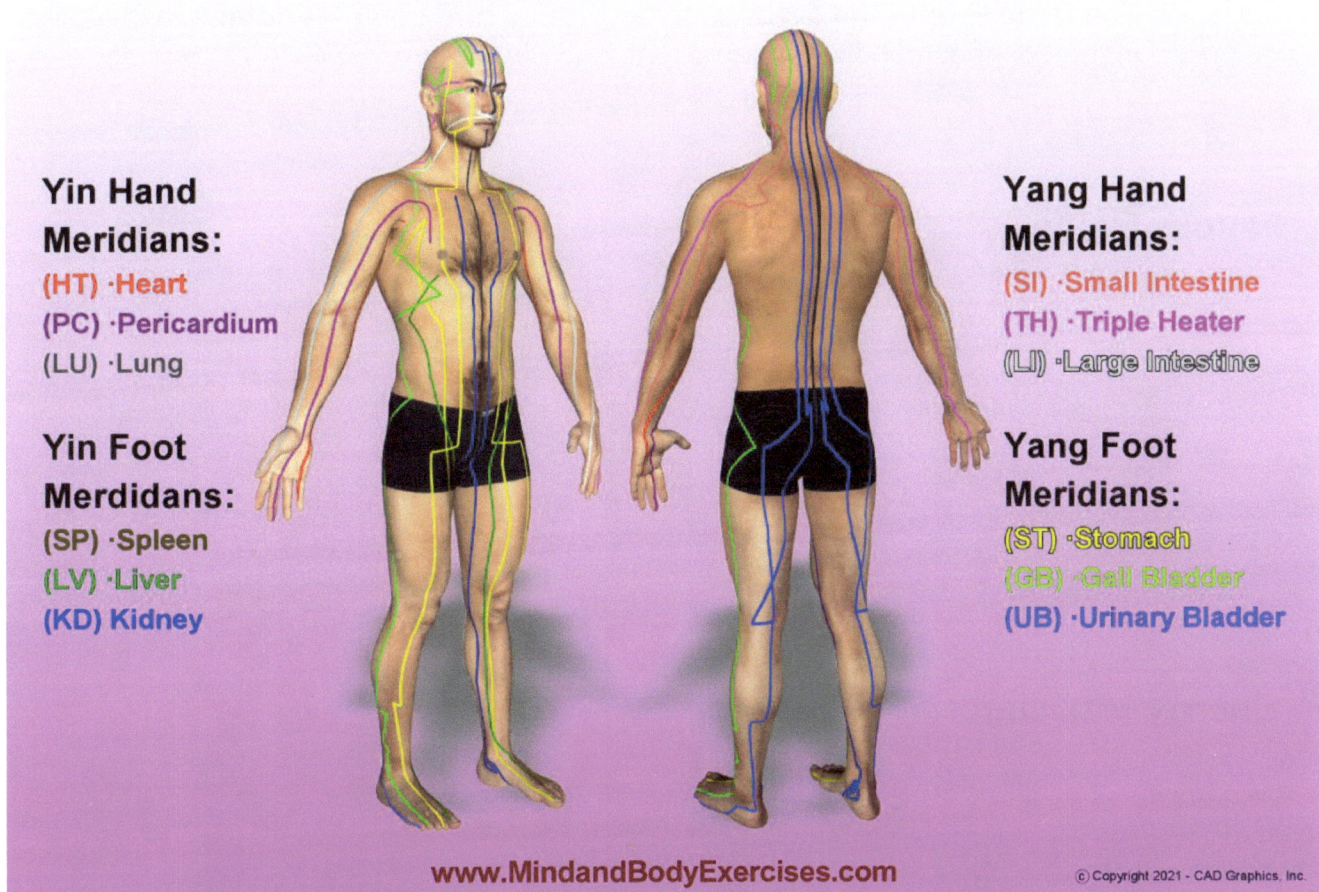

Yin Hand Meridians:
(HT) ·Heart
(PC) ·Pericardium
(LU) ·Lung

Yin Foot Merdidans:
(SP) ·Spleen
(LV) ·Liver
(KD) Kidney

Yang Hand Meridians:
(SI) ·Small Intestine
(TH) ·Triple Heater
(LI) ·Large Intestine

Yang Foot Meridians:
(ST) ·Stomach
(GB) ·Gall Bladder
(UB) ·Urinary Bladder

www.MindandBodyExercises.com

© Copyright 2021 - CAD Graphics, Inc.

1. Structural Similarities

- **Meridians in TCM** - In TCM, meridians are pathways through which **qi** (vital energy) flows, connecting organs, tissues, and systems. These pathways follow predictable routes along the body and influence both physical and energetic health.

- **Myofascial Trains -** Myofascial trains, as described by Myers, are continuous lines of fascia and connective tissue that transmit tension, force, and movement throughout the body. Myers identified 12 major myofascial lines, many of which mirror the flow of energy described by TCM meridians.

  Overlap: Many of the fascial lines align quite well with the primary TCM meridians:
  - The **Superficial Back Line** aligns with the **Bladder Meridian** running down the back.

  - The **Superficial Front Line** aligns the **Stomach and Spleen Meridians**.

- The **Lateral Line** aligns with the **Gallbladder Meridian**.

- The **Deep Front Line** aligns with the **Kidney and Liver Meridians**, especially in the connection between the psoas and diaphragm.

Fascia Trains

Superficial Front Line | Superficial Back Line | Spiral Line | Lateral Line | Deep Front Line | Superficial Front Arm Line | Deep Front Arm Line | Deep Back Arm Line | Superficial Back Arm Line

Energy Meridians

Stomach Meridian | Bladder Meridian | Stomach & Bladder Meridian | Gall Bladder Meridian | Kidney & Liver Meridian | Pericardium Meridian | Lung Meridian | Small Intestine Meridian | Triple Burner Meridian

www.MindAndBodyExercises.com

© Copyright 2018 - CAD Graphics, Inc.

2. Fascia's High-Water Content and Conductivity

- **Hydrophilic Nature:** Fascia is composed primarily of collagen and elastin fibers suspended in a gel-like ground substance known as the extracellular matrix (ECM), which is about 70-80% water. This high-water content allows fascia to conduct electrical signals efficiently.

- **Structured Water and Bioelectricity:** Within the fascia, water exists in a structured or "exclusion zone" (EZ) state, where the water molecules align in a crystalline lattice.

This structured water behaves like a semi-conductor, facilitating the transmission of bioelectric signals, which closely parallels the movement of *qi* in TCM.

- **Fascia's Role** - Fascia is highly innervated and acts as a communication network, responding to mechanical, chemical, and energetic stimuli. It conducts bioelectricity, making it a potential medium for the flow of *qi*.

- **Piezoelectric Effect** - When fascia is stretched or moved, it generates electrical charges through the piezoelectric effect. This phenomenon may correspond to the concept of qi moving through the meridians, providing a scientific basis for the energetic flow described in TCM.

3. Points of Intersection

- **Acupuncture Points and Fascial Crossroads** - Many acupuncture points are located where fascial planes intersect or where fascia connects with nerves, vessels, and muscles. Stimulating these points may influence both the fascia and the flow of energy, restoring balance in structure and energy flow

- **Trigger Points and *Ashi* Points** - rigger points in fascia often correspond to **Ashi points** in TCM. This overlap highlights a deep connection between fascial dysfunction and energy stagnation, further supporting the integration of these systems.

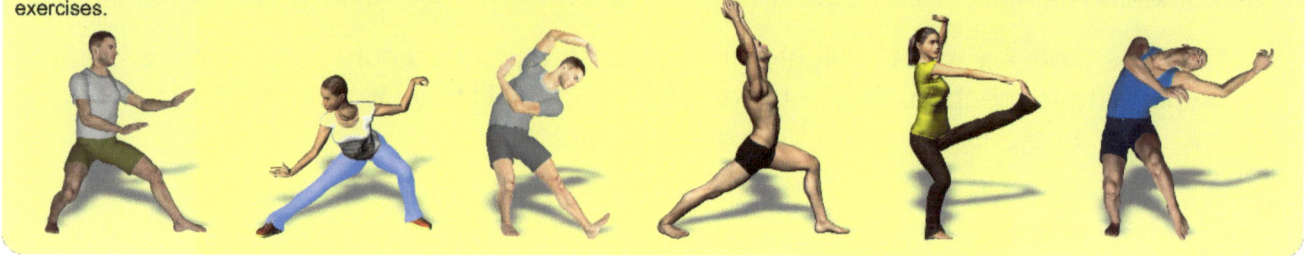

There are many individual exercises and techniques, that can stretch and release tension of the fascia trains throughout the human body. Tai Chi, Qigong, Yoga and Pilates are methods of stretching and strengthening the fascia as preventative or post-injury low impact exercises.

4. Dynamic Interplay of Movement and Energy

- **Tai Chi, Dao Yin and Qigong -** Practices like dao yin and Qigong manipulate both fascial tension and qi circulation, encouraging smooth flow along these pathways. The slow, mindful stretching and holding in these exercises release fascial restrictions while restoring balance to the meridians.

5. Scientific Validation Growing
- Studies using fMRI and infrared thermography have shown that needling acupuncture points activate areas along predictable pathways, which often align with fascial lines.

Research on fascia's bioelectric properties suggests that it may serve as the "physical" counterpart to the meridian system described in ancient texts. This growing body of evidence bridges the gap between TCM and modern anatomy

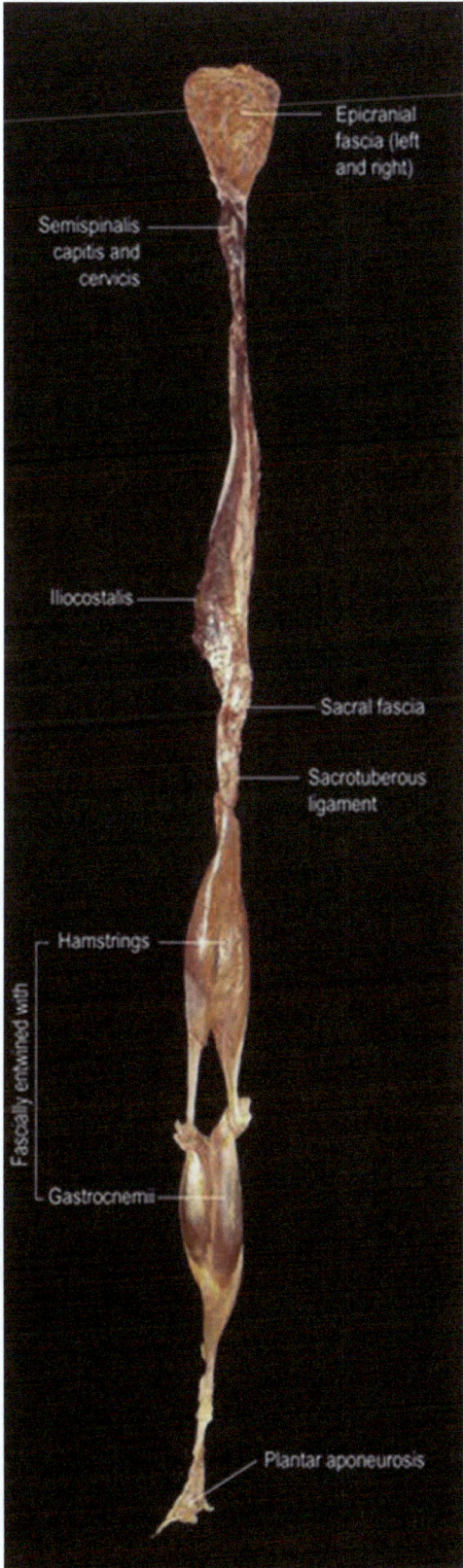

Epicranial fascia (left and right)

Semispinalis capitis and cervicis

Iliocostalis

Sacral fascia

Sacrotuberous ligament

Hamstrings

Fascially entwined with

Gastrocnemii

Plantar aponeurosis

A

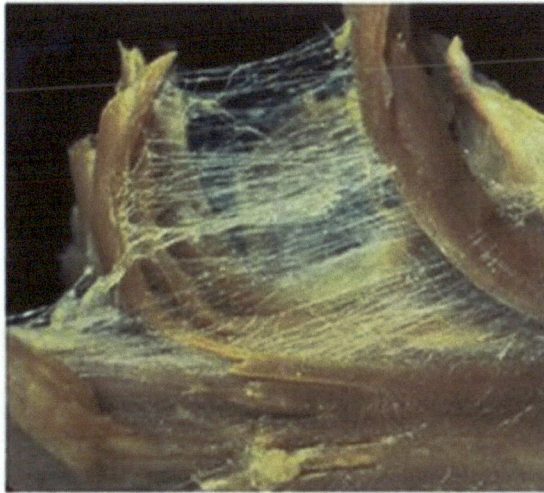

B

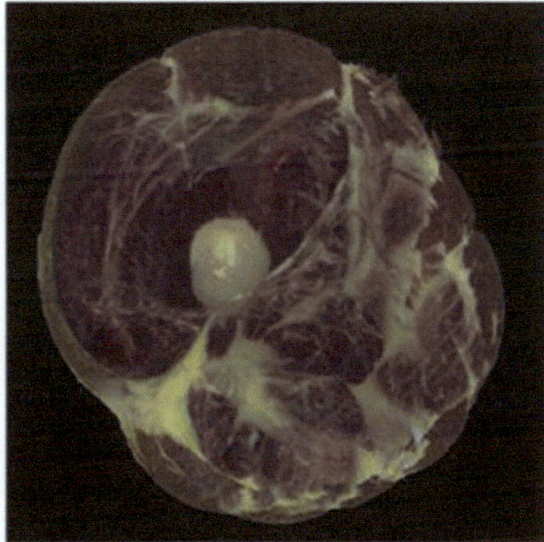

C

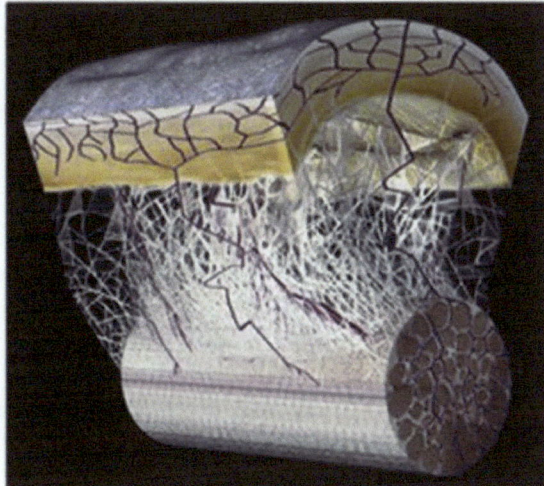

D

(Themes 2016)

85

5. Potential Implications

- **Holistic Therapies**

Combining myofascial release with acupressure or acupuncture can enhance therapeutic outcomes by addressing both the structural and energetic dimensions of the body. This integrated approach allows practitioners to work more holistically, benefiting patients on multiple levels.

- **Blending Ancient and Modern Knowledge**

Understanding the correlation between fascia and meridians helps modern therapists—such as osteopaths, physiotherapists, and acupuncturists apply ancient wisdom in a contemporary context. This connection exemplifies how ancient practices anticipated discoveries that Western science is only beginning to explore. In essence, fascia may serve as the physical matrix through which the meridian system operates, blending ancient wisdom with modern anatomy. This connection is a prime example of how ancient practices anticipated discoveries that Western science is just beginning to explore.

Fascia may serve as the physical matrix through which the meridian system operates, blending ancient TCM principles with modern anatomical insights. This evolving understanding highlights the profound interplay between structure and energy, offering a unified perspective on health and healing.

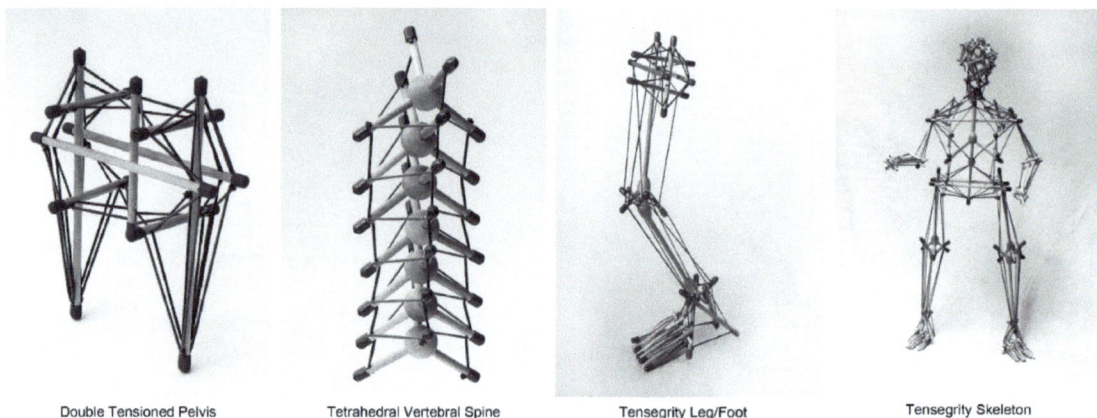

Double Tensioned Pelvis   Tetrahedral Vertebral Spine   Tensegrity Leg/Foot   Tensegrity Skeleton

References:

Myers, T. W. (2020). *Anatomy trains: Myofascial meridians for manual and movement therapists* (4th ed.). Elsevier.

Themes, U. (2016, June 11). *Fascia and biomechanical regulation*. Basicmedical Key. https://basicmedicalkey.com/fascia-and-biomechanical-regulation/

Yunshan, L., Chengli, X., Peiming, Z., Haocheng, Q., Xudong, L., & Liming, L. (2025). Integrative research on the mechanisms of acupuncture mechanics and interdisciplinary innovation. *BioMedical Engineering OnLine, 24*(1), 1–24. https://doi.org/10.1186/s12938-025-01357-w

In 1314, at the age of 71, Chen Wangting (or Chen Sheng Feng, as sometimes referenced in folklore) is said to have moved to Wudang Mountain. Inspired by an intense encounter between a snake and a bird, he observed how softness could overcome hardness and how yielding could neutralize force. Combining the deadly precision of their movements with his extensive knowledge of military Longfist (Changquan) techniques, he began to refine his martial practice.

To this foundation, he integrated:

- **The dynamic interplay of Yin and Yang**, expressing the natural balance of opposing forces.

- **The Five Element (Wu Xing) energy movements** of ancient Taoists.

- **Ancient Dao Yin exercises**, promoting internal health and longevity.

- **The environmental harmony of the I Ching** emphasizing adaptability and flow.

- **The philosophy of the Tao Te Ching**, guiding the practitioner toward a path of spiritual harmony and natural wisdom.

This synthesis evolved into what became known as **Tai Chi Chuan (Taijiquan or "supreme ultimate fist")**, later branching into the Five Element Tai Chi system.
Tai Chi can be likened to:

- **A doctor**, as it promotes healing and internal balance.

- **A soldier**, as it is an effective method of self-defense.

- **Vitality for the elderly** and **focus for the young.**

It is an exercise that strengthens the body, a meditation that calms the mind, a combat system that trains awareness and control, and a path of personal development that leads to deeper understanding. Tai Chi is like yoga in its pursuit of flexibility and balance, like dance in its graceful movements, and like self-defense in its strategic applications.

Ultimately, Tai Chi seeks to cultivate harmony with nature, instill discipline through spirituality, foster health and resilience in the individual, and align one's being with the heavens. It is hundreds of years old, a living expression of the Dao—the Way of Tai Chi Chuan.

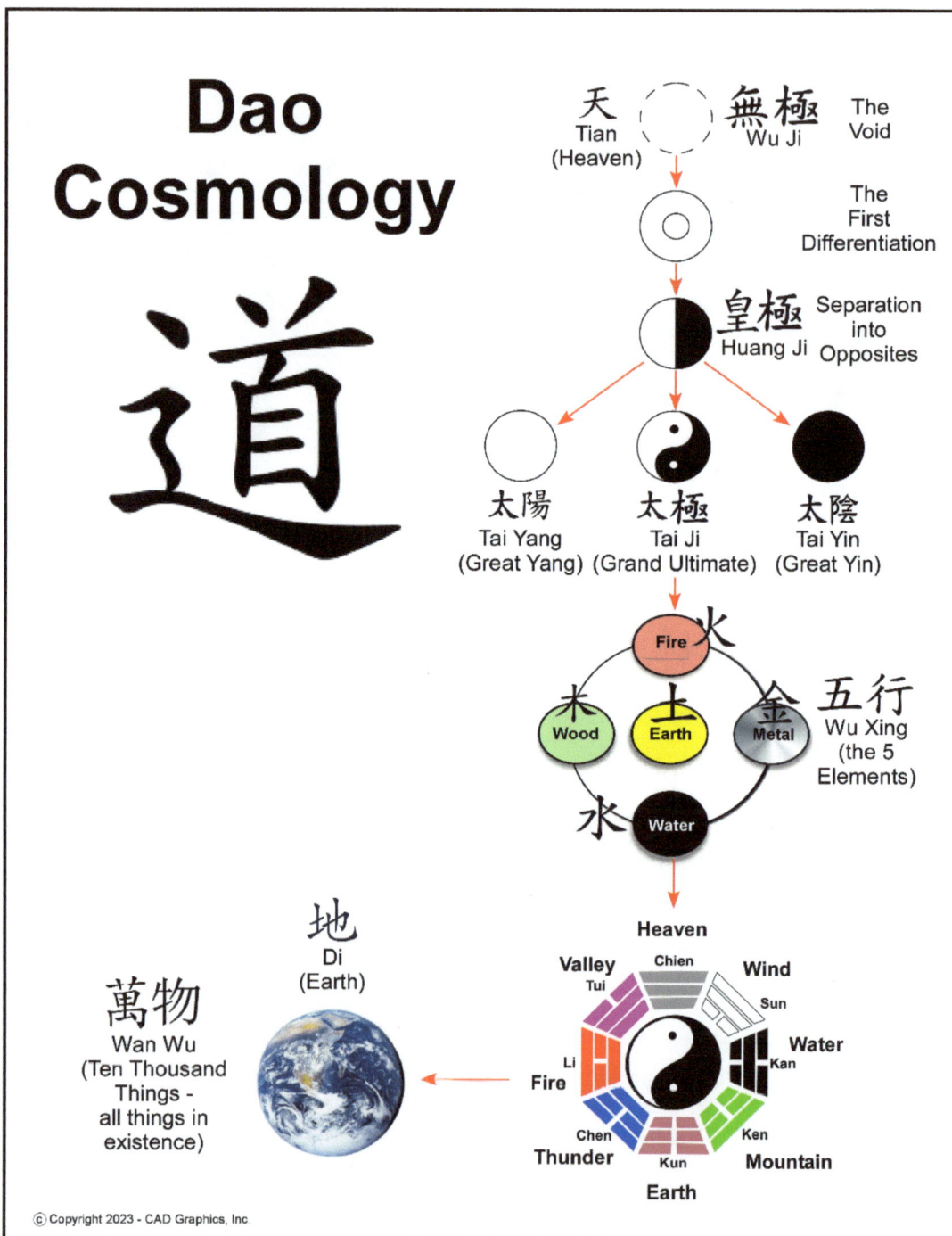

© Copyright 2023 - CAD Graphics, Inc.

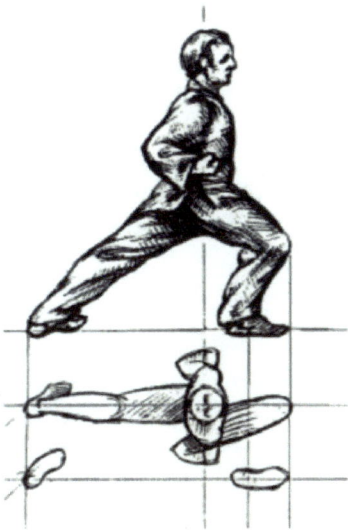

Bow and Arrow

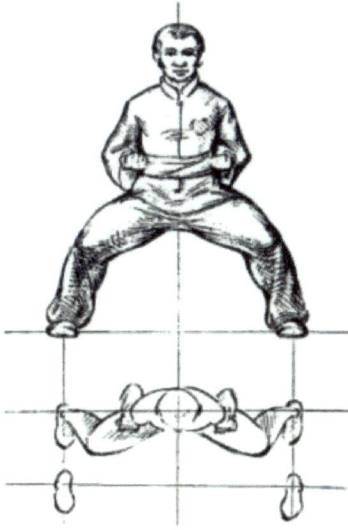

Horse Stance

L or Half Horse

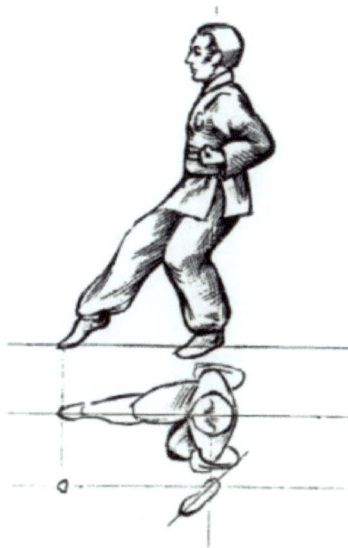

Empty

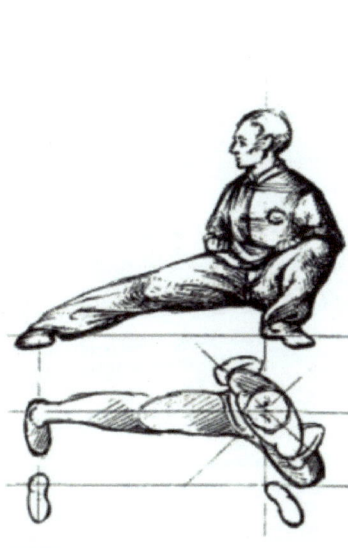

Tiger

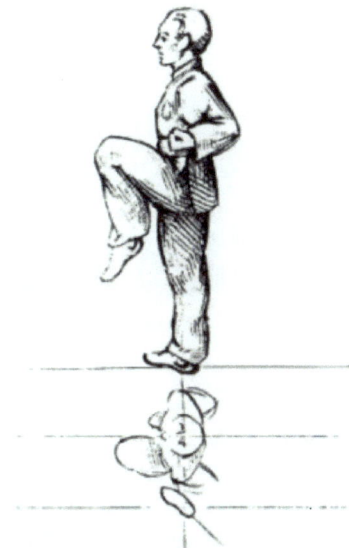

Rooster

Art Work: Guy Robinson of Atlanta, Georgia

What Is Autogenic Therapy? A Self-Directed Path to Deep Relaxation

In today's fast-paced world, stress-related conditions are on the rise. Autogenic therapy, also known as **autogenic training,** offers a powerful way to counterbalance modern stress through a simple, structured set of mental exercises. Developed by German psychiatrist Johannes Heinrich Schultz in the early 20th century, this self-regulation technique continues to help people worldwide regain calm, reduce anxiety, and improve overall well-being (VA Office of Patient Centered Care and Cultural Transformation, n.d.)

What Is Autogenic Therapy?

Autogenic therapy is a relaxation technique that uses self-suggestions to bring about physical and emotional calmness. The practice involves six standardized exercises focusing on sensations like:

- Heaviness and lightness in the limbs
- Warmth
- Heartbeat regulation
- Breathing awareness
- Abdominal warmth
- Forehead cooling (Luthe & Schultz, 1969)

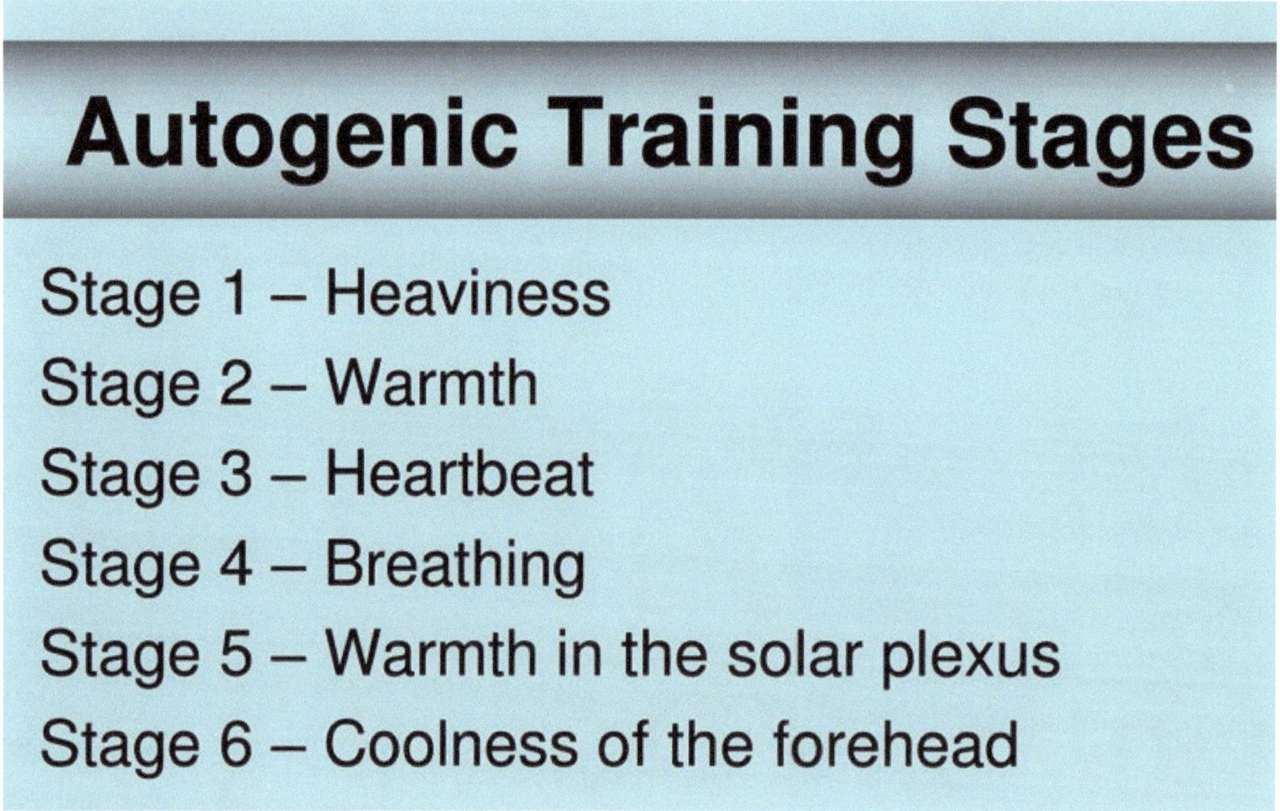

Autogenic Training Stages
Stage 1 – Heaviness
Stage 2 – Warmth
Stage 3 – Heartbeat
Stage 4 – Breathing
Stage 5 – Warmth in the solar plexus
Stage 6 – Coolness of the forehead

These exercises promote a shift in the autonomic nervous system toward the parasympathetic or *"rest and digest"* mode, reducing the physiological effects of stress.

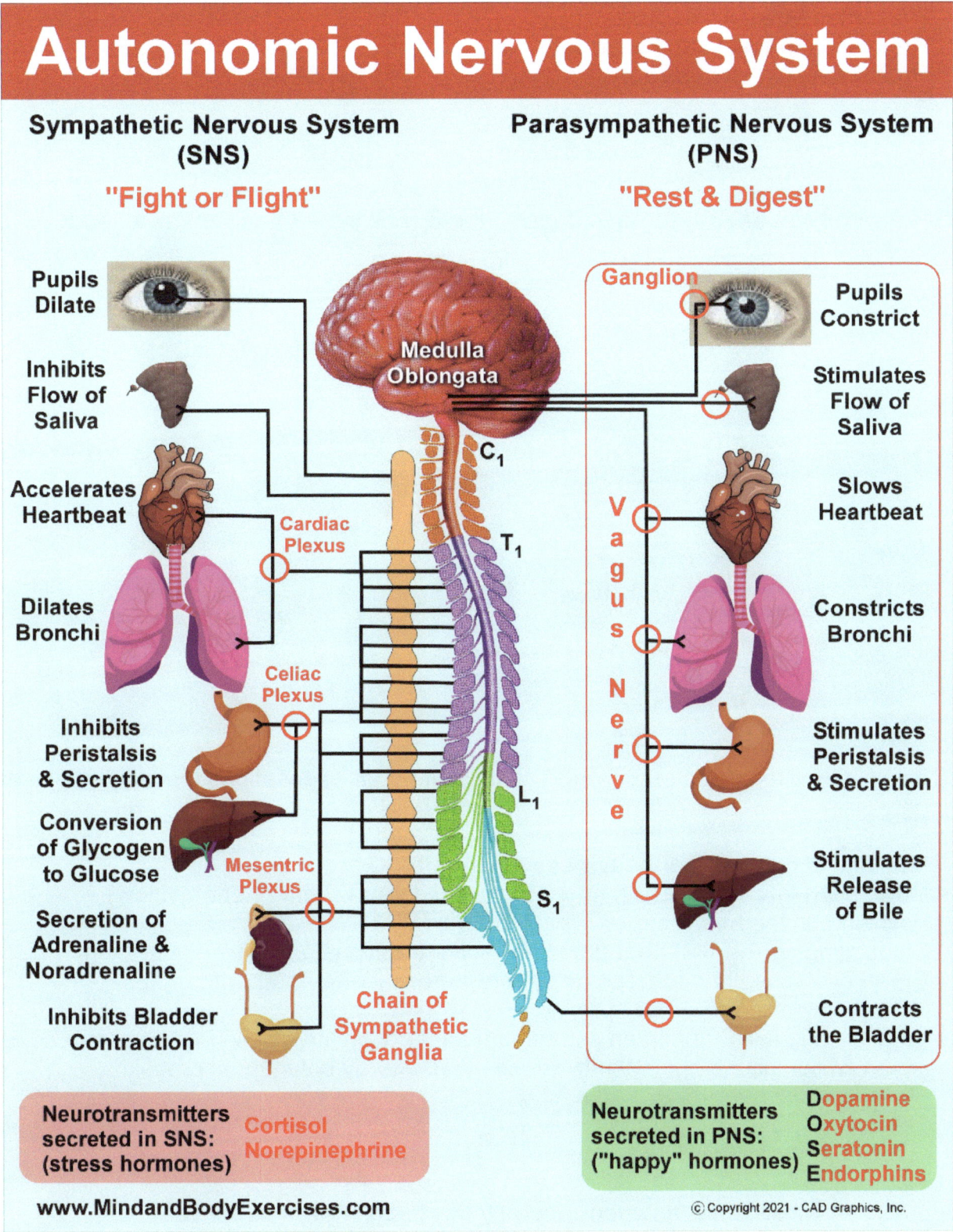

Autonomic Nervous System

Sympathetic Nervous System (SNS)

"Fight or Flight"

Pupils Dilate

Inhibits Flow of Saliva

Accelerates Heartbeat

Cardiac Plexus

Dilates Bronchi

Celiac Plexus

Inhibits Peristalsis & Secretion

Conversion of Glycogen to Glucose

Mesentric Plexus

Secretion of Adrenaline & Noradrenaline

Inhibits Bladder Contraction

Chain of Sympathetic Ganglia

Medulla Oblongata

C_1

T_1

L_1

S_1

Parasympathetic Nervous System (PNS)

"Rest & Digest"

Ganglion

Pupils Constrict

Stimulates Flow of Saliva

Slows Heartbeat

Vagus Nerve

Constricts Bronchi

Stimulates Peristalsis & Secretion

Stimulates Release of Bile

Contracts the Bladder

Neurotransmitters secreted in SNS: (stress hormones) — Cortisol, Norepinephrine

Neurotransmitters secreted in PNS: ("happy" hormones) — Dopamine, Oxytocin, Seratonin, Endorphins

www.MindandBodyExercises.com

© Copyright 2021 - CAD Graphics, Inc.

Although not usually classified as meditation, autogenic therapy shares similar traits with meditative and mindfulness-based practices:

- Present-moment awareness
- Regulation of breath and heart rate
- Promotion of internal balance and nervous system calm (Melnikov, 2021)

A Shared Language: Body Awareness in Mind–Body Disciplines

What's especially fascinating is that autogenic therapy aligns with ancient mind–body traditions found in:

- Tai Chi
- Qigong
- Yoga
- Martial Arts

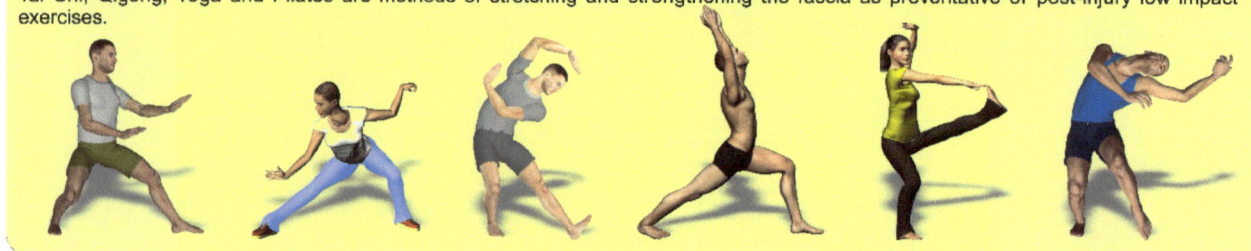

There are many individual exercises and techniques, that can stretch and release tension of the fascia trains throughout the human body. Tai Chi, Qigong, Yoga and Pilates are methods of stretching and strengthening the fascia as preventative or post-injury low impact exercises.

These disciplines often guide practitioners to cultivate bodily sensations that echo those used in autogenic training:

- Feelings of **lightness** or **heaviness** in the limbs
- Generating **internal warmth** (often associated with breath or energy flow)
- Focusing on the **heartbeat** or **breath rhythm**
- Stimulating **abdominal heat** (known in some traditions as *dantian* activation)
- Creating a sense of **coolness or spaciousness** in the head or forehead

These parallels suggest that human self-regulation, through structured inner awareness, is a timeless and cross-cultural approach to stress relief, energy balance, and health.

Benefits of Autogenic Training

When practiced consistently, autogenic therapy has been shown to:

- Reduce anxiety and stress
- Improve sleep quality
- Lower blood pressure
- Enhance emotional and nervous system resilience
- Relieve headaches, muscle tension, and chronic fatigue (Stetter & Kupper, 2002)

Its simplicity and accessibility make it a popular choice for those looking for holistic, non-invasive ways to manage daily pressures and improve health.

How It Works

Each autogenic session involves repeating mental phrases such as, "my arms are heavy and warm," while reclining or sitting in a quiet space. The mind's focus on these specific body cues leads to a measurable shift in physiology, lowering stress hormones, heart rate, and muscle tension (Luthe & Schultz, 1969; Stetter & Kupper, 2002).

Many people practice autogenic training independently, with audio guidance, or under the supervision of a certified therapist.

⚠ Caution: Autogenic Training and Psychotic Disorders

While autogenic therapy is safe for most individuals, it may not be appropriate for people with psychotic disorders, such as schizophrenia or bipolar disorder with psychotic features (Fletcher, 2023). Here's why:

1. Exacerbation of Symptoms

The use of self-suggestion and imagery can potentially worsen hallucinations or delusional thinking in vulnerable individuals (Stetter & Kupper, 2002).

2. Potential for Dissociation

The deep relaxation states achieved may induce altered consciousness or dissociation, which can be unsettling or unsafe for those with psychotic tendencies.

3. Difficulty in Reality Testing

Psychotic conditions often impair one's ability to distinguish between internal experience and external reality. Autogenic training might blur these lines further (Stetter & Kupper, 2002).

4. Medication Disruption Risk

Some individuals may believe that relaxation practices can replace essential medication, potentially leading to non-compliance and relapses (Mueser & Jeste, 2008)

Because of these risks, it's essential that individuals with psychotic disorders engage in any form of relaxation training only under professional medical supervision. More recent research has suggested that autogenic therapy may actually help those suffering from schizophrenia (Breznoscakova et al., 2023).

Final Thoughts

Autogenic therapy offers a safe, evidence-based, and self-directed method to reduce stress and promote relaxation. Its emphasis on internal sensations such as warmth, breath, heartbeat, and mental stillness, places it in harmony with long-standing Eastern practices like tai chi, yoga, and qigong.

For most people, autogenic therapy can serve as a cornerstone of a healthy lifestyle, but those with complex mental health conditions should consult with trained professionals to ensure it is suitable.

References:

Breznoscakova, D., Kovanicova, M., Sedlakova, E., & Pallayova, M. (2023). Autogenic Training in Mental Disorders: What Can We Expect? *International Journal of Environmental Research and Public Health*, *20*(5), 4344. https://doi.org/10.3390/ijerph20054344

Fletcher, J. (2023, August 17). *Autogenic training: Benefits, limitations, and how to do it*. https://www.medicalnewstoday.com/articles/autogenic-training#how-to-do-it

Luthe, W., & Schultz, J. H. (1969). *Autogenic therapy* (Vol. 1–6). New York: Grune & Stratton. Mueser, K. T., & Jeste, D. V. (2008). *Clinical handbook of schizophrenia*. New York: Guilford Press.

Melnikov, M. Y. (2021). The Current Evidence Levels for Biofeedback and Neurofeedback Interventions in Treating Depression: A Narrative review. *Neural Plasticity*, *2021*, 1–31. https://doi.org/10.1155/2021/8878857

Stetter, F., & Kupper, S. (2002). Autogenic training: a meta-analysis of clinical outcome studies. *Applied Psychophysiology and Biofeedback*, *27*(1), 45–98. https://doi.org/10.1023/a:1014576505223

VA Office of Patient Centered Care and Cultural Transformation. (n.d.). AUTOGENIC TRAINING. In *VA Office of Patient Centered Care and Cultural Transformation* (pp. 1–3). https://www.va.gov/WHOLEHEALTHLIBRARY/docs/Autogenic-Training.pdf

The Interconnectedness of Physical Fitness Aspects

The many facets of fitness can be prioritized depending on individual goals and needs. Below is a list of key fitness components, with explanations of how and why each is important, and their order of prioritization based on general health, athletic performance, and functional movement.

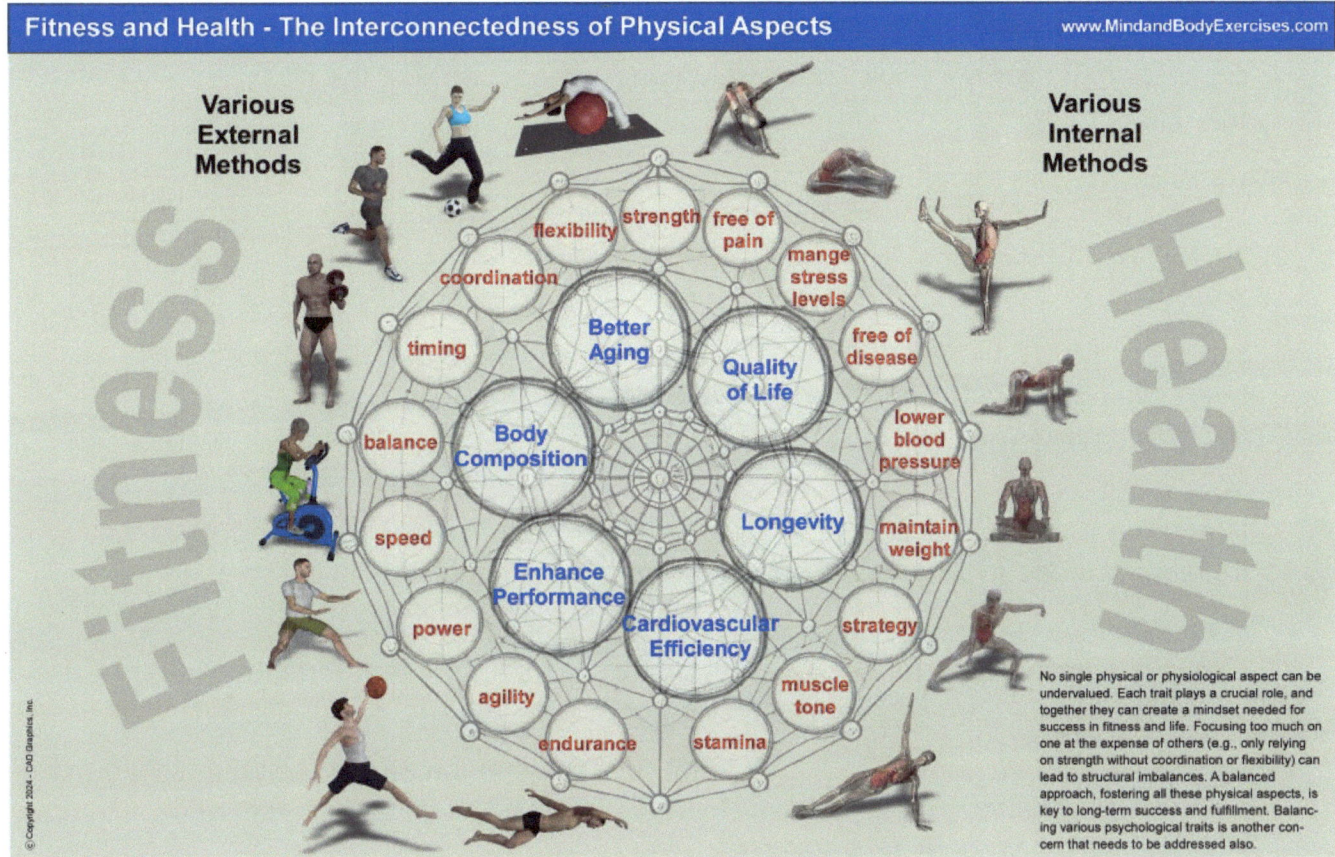

Fitness and Health - The Interconnectedness of Physical Aspects   www.MindandBodyExercises.com

Various External Methods

Various Internal Methods

flexibility · strength · free of pain · mange stress levels · coordination · Better Aging · free of disease · timing · Quality of Life · balance · Body Composition · lower blood pressure · speed · Longevity · maintain weight · Enhance Performance · power · Cardiovascular Efficiency · strategy · agility · muscle tone · endurance · stamina

No single physical or physiological aspect can be undervalued. Each trait plays a crucial role, and together they can create a mindset needed for success in fitness and life. Focusing too much on one at the expense of others (e.g., only relying on strength without coordination or flexibility) can lead to structural imbalances. A balanced approach, fostering all these physical aspects, is key to long-term success and fulfillment. Balancing various psychological traits is another concern that needs to be addressed also.

1. Strength
- **How:** The ability of muscles to exert force. Strength is developed through resistance training, such as weightlifting or bodyweight exercises.

- **Why:** Strength forms the foundation for most physical activities. It supports bone health, maintains muscle mass, aids in balance, and helps prevent injury by stabilizing joints and improving posture.

2. Flexibility
- **How:** The range of motion around a joint or group of joints. Flexibility is improved through stretching exercises (static, dynamic, or PNF (Proprioceptive Neuromuscular Facilitation).

95

- **Why:** Flexibility helps prevent injury by allowing muscles to move more freely. It supports overall mobility, reduces muscle stiffness, and aids in the recovery process. It's essential for maintaining functional movement, especially as we age.

3. Coordination
- **How:** The ability to synchronize multiple body movements smoothly and efficiently. Coordination can be developed through balance exercises, agility drills, or sports.

- **Why:** Coordination is crucial for functional fitness, sports performance, and injury prevention. It allows for fluid movements and better control of the body in daily activities.

4. Endurance (Cardiovascular)
- **How:** The ability of the heart and lungs to deliver oxygen to working muscles during sustained physical activity. It's improved through aerobic exercises like running, swimming, or cycling.

- **Why:** Cardiovascular endurance is vital for overall health. It helps lower the risk of heart disease, boosts energy levels, and enhances the body's ability to perform sustained tasks with less fatigue.

5. Balance
- **How:** The ability to maintain body position while standing still or moving. Balance training includes exercises like yoga, Tai Chi, or standing on one leg.

- **Why:** Balance is especially important for functional fitness and preventing falls, particularly as we age. It also supports better posture and coordination.

6. Power
- **How:** The ability to exert a maximal amount of force in the shortest possible time (a combination of strength and speed). Power is developed through plyometrics, Olympic lifts, and explosive body movements.

- **Why:** Power is crucial for activities requiring quick, explosive movements such as sprinting or jumping. It's key for athletes but also benefits functional movement by improving reaction time and performance in high-intensity tasks.

7. Speed
- **How:** The ability to move quickly in a specific direction. Speed can be enhanced through sprint training, interval workouts, and agility drills.

- **Why:** Speed is critical for athletic performance but also useful in daily life for tasks that require quick movement or reaction, such as running after a bus or responding to emergencies.

8. Agility
- **How:** The ability to change direction quickly and efficiently. Agility training often involves cone drills, ladder drills, and quick lateral movements.

- **Why:** Agility is essential for athletes in sports that require fast directional changes. It also benefits non-athletes by improving body control and reducing injury risks during dynamic activities.

9. Timing
- **How:** The ability to move or react at the right moment. Timing is often developed through sports, reaction drills, or coordination exercises.

- **Why:** Good timing enhances coordination and athletic performance, particularly in sports like tennis, boxing, or baseball where precision is key.

10. Control
- **How:** The ability to regulate and maintain body position and movement. Control is improved through strength, balance, and proprioception exercises.

- **Why:** Control is necessary for mastering technique in physical activities. It enhances precision, reduces the risk of injury, and helps in maintaining stability and proper form during movements.

11. Reaction Time
- **How:** The speed at which an individual can respond to a stimulus. Reaction time can be improved through drills involving quick decision-making or unexpected changes.

- **Why:** Faster reaction time is beneficial for safety and athletic performance, allowing a quicker response to environmental changes or dynamic sports scenarios.

Prioritization Based on Goals:

1. **For General Health and Longevity:**
   - Strength, Flexibility, Endurance, Balance
     - These components promote muscle and bone health, reduce injury risk, and improve heart health and mobility, all crucial for everyday functionality.

2. **For Athletic Performance:**
   - Power, Speed, Agility, Coordination, Endurance
     - Athletes benefit most from power and agility to enhance performance in sports, where explosive movements and quick reactions are needed.

3. **For Functional Fitness and Injury Prevention:**
   - Balance, Coordination, Strength, Control, Timing
     - These aspects ensure better stability, posture, and fluid movements, which are essential for performing daily tasks and preventing accidents.

Each component of fitness is interrelated and essential for a well-rounded approach to health and performance. Prioritization should be tailored to personal goals, whether that's improving overall health, preparing for sports, or maintaining functional mobility as we age. We really can't state that one aspect is most important, such as balance, which, if someone has none, cannot achieve the others. Or without coordination, one cannot develop more strength or more flexibility, correct? Or without strength, there is no balance to stabilize? All are important and cannot be underprioritized, correct?

The various facets of fitness are interconnected, and it's difficult to isolate one as the most important because they all support and influence each other.

- **Balance** is essential for safe and effective movement, but it often requires a certain amount of strength and coordination to maintain.

- **Strength** helps with balance and supports mobility, but flexibility is needed to allow the muscles and joints to move freely.

- **Coordination** is necessary to execute movements smoothly, but strength and timing also influence how well we can control those movements.

In essence, none of these components can be fully developed in isolation. Each contributes to overall fitness and functional capacity, so under-prioritizing any one of them could limit progress in other areas. It's important to approach fitness in a holistic way, ensuring that all aspects are integrated and developed according to personal goals and needs.

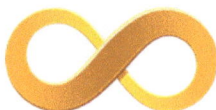

Psychological Aspects of Fitness are as Interconnected as the Physical Components

Mental and psychological aspects of fitness are as interconnected as the physical components. Each plays a crucial role in supporting not only physical training but overall well-being. Let's look at these mental attributes in the context of fitness training, their importance, and how they influence one another.

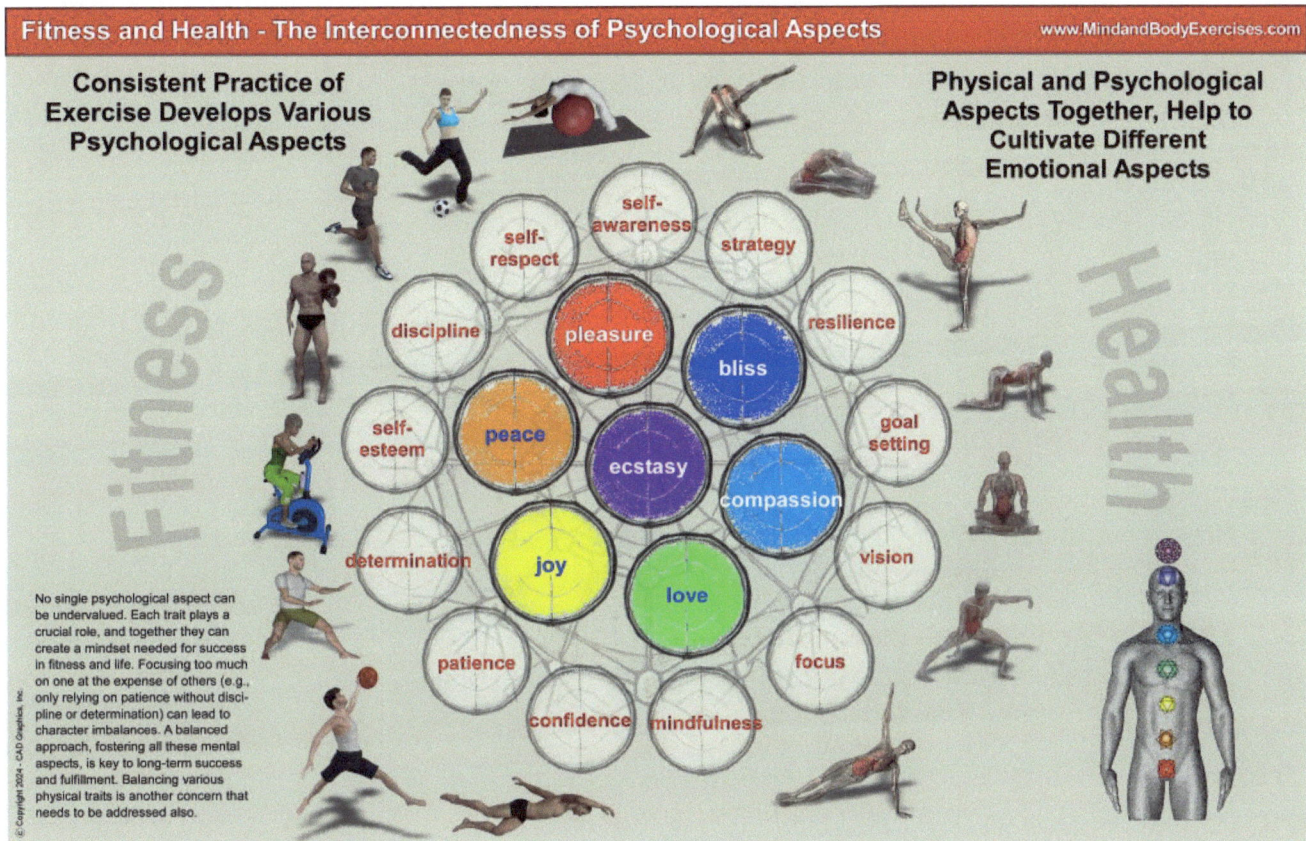

Fitness and Health - The Interconnectedness of Psychological Aspects — www.MindandBodyExercises.com

1. Determination (Perseverance)
- **How:** The ability to stick with a fitness routine and push through challenges, even when motivation wanes.

- **Why:** Determination is essential for achieving long-term goals. It's the driving force that helps you overcome obstacles like fatigue, frustration, or setbacks. Without it, progress stalls when the going gets tough.

2. Focus
- **How:** The ability to concentrate on a specific task, whether it's executing proper form during an exercise or staying on track with fitness goals.

- **Why:** Focus is critical for making the most of workouts and for avoiding distractions that can hinder progress. It ensures that you give your best effort, improving both efficiency and performance during training.

3. Confidence
- **How:** Belief in your own ability to succeed, whether in reaching fitness milestones or mastering a new skill.

- **Why:** Confidence is key for pushing boundaries and trying new things. It helps you trust in your physical capabilities, which in turn supports better performance and a more positive experience with exercise. Confidence grows as you achieve goals, fueling further progress.

4. Self-Esteem
- **How:** The overall sense of self-worth or value, often influenced by body image, fitness achievements, and general well-being.

- **Why:** Self-esteem is closely tied to mental health and motivation. People with healthy self-esteem are more likely to stick to their fitness routines because they feel good about their efforts and outcomes. Low self-esteem, on the other hand, can lead to negative thinking patterns, discouraging progress.

5. Resilience
- **How:** The ability to recover quickly from setbacks, whether it's a physical injury or a period of demotivation.

- **Why:** Resilience helps you bounce back from failures or obstacles without giving up. In fitness, this means returning to your program after illness, injury, or emotional challenges, rather than letting those issues derail progress.

6. Discipline
- **How:** The ability to maintain consistency with workouts, nutrition, and recovery, even when it's not easy or convenient.

- **Why:** Discipline is foundational to any fitness journey. It bridges the gap between intention and action, helping you stick to your program even when motivation fades. Without discipline, fitness goals are harder to achieve because they require sustained effort over time.

7. Patience
- **How:** The ability to recognize that results take time and to persist without frustration or rushing the process.

- **Why:** Patience is critical for long-term success. Fitness gains often come slowly, and without patience, it's easy to get discouraged or try to fast-track results, which can lead to injury or burnout.

8. Self-Awareness

- **How:** The ability to assess your own thoughts, emotions, and behaviors in relation to fitness goals and progress.

- **Why:** Self-awareness helps you understand your limits, strengths, and areas for improvement. It's essential for setting realistic goals, avoiding overtraining, and recognizing when adjustments need to be made in your routine.

9. Mindfulness

- **How:** The ability to be fully present and engaged in the current moment, whether during a workout or throughout the day.

- **Why:** Mindfulness enhances focus and reduces stress. When applied to fitness, it helps you connect with your body, prevent injuries, and make intentional choices in your movements. It also fosters a healthier relationship with exercise, avoiding compulsive behaviors.

10. Goal setting (Vision)

- **How:** The ability to establish clear, achievable objectives and a vision for where you want to go.

- **Why:** Without clear goals, it's easy to drift in your fitness journey. Goal setting provides direction, helps maintain motivation, and offers a sense of purpose in your efforts. It also gives a framework for measuring progress, which builds confidence and determination.

Interconnected Nature:

- **Determination** supports **discipline** and **resilience**; without it, it's hard to remain consistent through challenges.

- **Focus** helps improve **self-awareness** and **mindfulness**, allowing you to make better decisions during training.

- **Confidence** feeds into **self-esteem**, as success in fitness tasks increases self-worth and encourages further progress.

- **Patience** and **resilience** go hand-in-hand, ensuring that setbacks or slow progress do not deter long-term success.

- **Discipline** keeps you on track even when motivation wanes, ensuring that **patience** and **goal setting** are upheld.

Prioritization of Mental Aspects:

1. **For Sustained Progress:**

   - **Determination, Discipline, Focus, Patience**

     - These traits help ensure consistency in efforts, overcoming plateaus and sticking to long-term plans.

2. **For Building Confidence and Positive Self-Perception:**

   - **Self-Esteem, Resilience**

     - Developing confidence and self-esteem through small wins and resilience in the face of setbacks is essential for long-term mental well-being.

3. **For Better Daily Performance:**

   - **Focus, Mindfulness, Self-Awareness**

     - These help you stay present during workouts, manage stress, and stay aligned with your goals, ensuring efficiency and enjoyment in training.

Conclusion:

Just as with physical fitness, no single mental or psychological aspect can be undervalued. Each trait plays a crucial role, and together they create the mindset needed for success in fitness and life. Focusing too much on one at the expense of others (e.g., only relying on discipline without self-awareness or resilience) can lead to burnout or frustration. A balanced approach, fostering all these mental aspects, is key to long-term success and fulfillment.

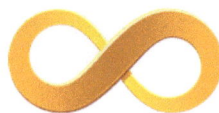

Wind and Water, Makes Fire

The human mind and body are integral parts of nature, constantly interacting with its energies. There is a direct correlation between the systems of nature and those of the body, with three key elements of wind, fire, and water, serving as points of connection.

- **Wind** corresponds to the respiratory system, as the air we breathe sustains life.

- **Fire** represents body temperature, which plays a vital role in all physiological functions.

- **Water** relates to the circulatory system, essential for vitality and well-being.

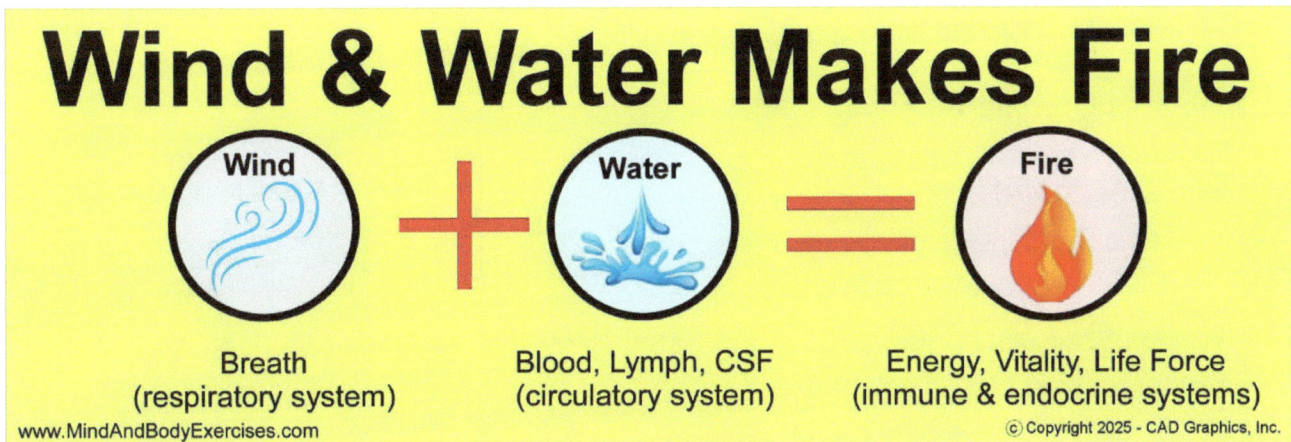

Wind & Water Makes Fire

Wind	Water	Fire
Breath (respiratory system)	Blood, Lymph, CSF (circulatory system)	Energy, Vitality, Life Force (immune & endocrine systems)

www.MindAndBodyExercises.com © Copyright 2025 - CAD Graphics, Inc.

Practices such as Tai Chi, Qigong, and Bagua Zhang profoundly influence the body, impacting the organs, joints, and muscles at a deep level. In Taoist alchemy, the philosophical phrase *"wind and water make fire"* metaphorically represents the dynamic interactions of the Five Elements (Wu Xing) and the internal processes of self-cultivation.

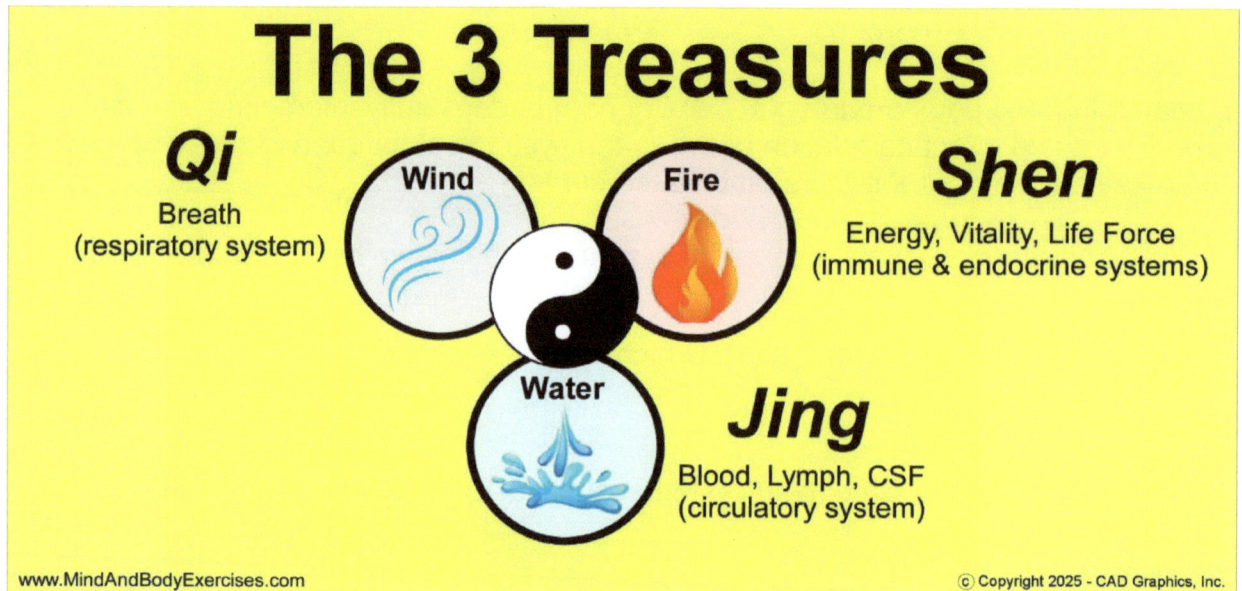

The 3 Treasures

Qi
Breath
(respiratory system)

Wind

Fire

Shen
Energy, Vitality, Life Force
(immune & endocrine systems)

Water

Jing
Blood, Lymph, CSF
(circulatory system)

www.MindAndBodyExercises.com

© Copyright 2025 - CAD Graphics, Inc.

Here's a breakdown of how this concept fits into Taoist thought:

Five Elements Correspondence:

- **Wind (Feng, 风)** is often associated with Wood (Mu, 木), which represents growth, movement, and expansion.

- **Water (Shui, 水)** corresponds to the Kidneys and the essence (Jing), which serves as the foundation for transformation.

- **Fire (Huo, 火)** corresponds to Yang energy, warmth, and spirit (Shen).

- The idea is that the interaction of movement (Wind/Wood) and nourishment (Water) can generate Fire (Yang energy, transformation).

Neidan (Internal Alchemy) Interpretation:

- Wind (Wood) and Water represent Qi and Jing, respectively.

- Their controlled interaction through breathwork, meditation, and energy circulation can generate the internal **"alchemy fire"** needed to refine essence into Qi and Qi into Shen.

- This fire is not literal but the internal warmth and energetic transformation that happens in deep meditation or Qigong.

Martial & Qigong Perspective:

- In advanced Qigong and martial arts, regulated breath (Wind) and internal fluid movement (Water) manifest into internal heat (Fire), leading to refined power and vitality.

- This aligns with practices of Tai Chi, Qigong and BaguaZhang, where breath, body movement, and mind-intent cultivate the internal fire for vitality and martial efficiency.

Wind & Water Makes Fire

Wind + Water = Fire

Breath
(respiratory system)

Blood, Lymph, CSF
(circulatory system)

Energy, Vitality, Life Force
(immune & endocrine systems)

風 **Wind**
baguazhang

水 **Water**
tai chi

火 **Fire**
qigong

each practice has components of wind, water & fire

www.MindAndBodyExercises.com

© Copyright 2025 - CAD Graphics, Inc.

SECTION IV: Mental Health, Awareness & Psychology

Key Neurotransmitters Involved in Mood Regulation

Neurotransmitters are chemical messengers within the brain that are essential in regulating mood, emotions, and overall mental health. These substances interact in complex ways to influence psychological well-being. Below are some of the principal neurotransmitters involved in mood regulation:

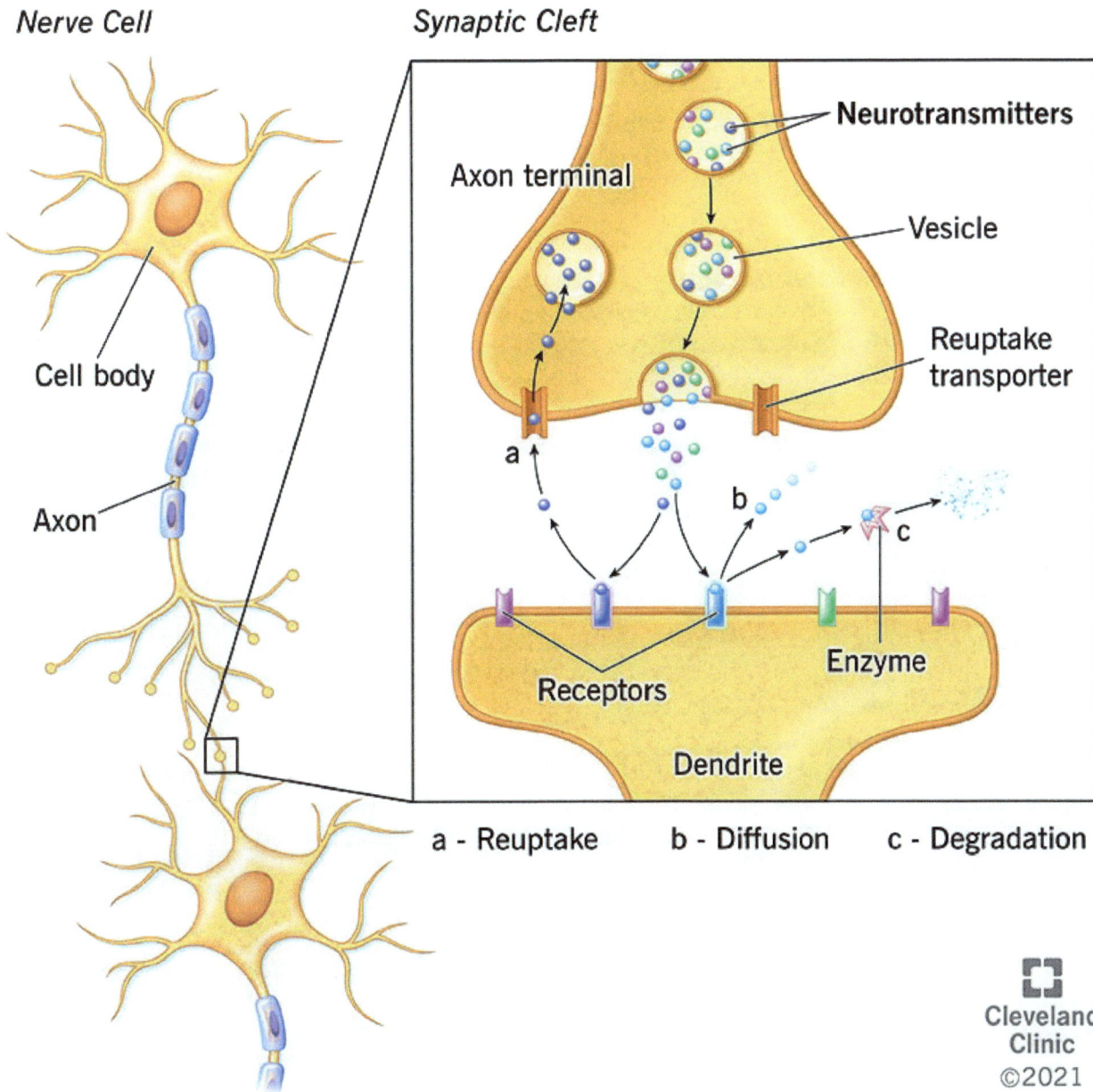

Nerve Cell

Synaptic Cleft

Neurotransmitters

Axon terminal

Vesicle

Reuptake transporter

Cell body

Axon

a

b

c

Receptors

Enzyme

Dendrite

a - Reuptake   b - Diffusion   c - Degradation

Cleveland Clinic
©2021

https://my.clevelandclinic.org/health/articles/22513-neurotransmitters

Serotonin (5-HT) – Often called the "feel-good" neurotransmitter, serotonin helps regulate mood, anxiety, sleep, appetite, and digestion. Low levels are linked to depression and anxiety disorders. Many antidepressants (SSRIs) work by increasing serotonin availability in the synaptic cleft, though the precise mechanism of their effect on mood is still being studied.

Dopamine (DA) – Associated with pleasure, motivation, and reward, dopamine reinforces positive behaviors and plays a key role in learning and movement. Low dopamine levels are linked to depression, lack of motivation, and anhedonia (inability to feel pleasure), while excessive dopamine activity in certain brain regions is associated with schizophrenia. It is also crucial for motor control, with deficiencies contributing to Parkinson's disease.

Norepinephrine (NE) – A neurotransmitter and stress hormone that regulates alertness, energy, and the body's "fight or flight" response. Low levels are associated with depression and fatigue, while high levels can contribute to anxiety, hypervigilance, and increased heart rate. Some antidepressants (SNRIs and tricyclics) work by increasing norepinephrine availability.

GABA (Gamma-Aminobutyric Acid) – The primary inhibitory neurotransmitter, GABA helps calm brain activity and reduce stress and anxiety. Low GABA levels are linked to anxiety disorders, insomnia, and epilepsy. Substances like benzodiazepines and alcohol enhance GABA's effects, leading to their sedative and anti-anxiety properties.

Glutamate – The brain's primary excitatory neurotransmitter, glutamate is essential for learning, memory, and cognitive function. However, excessive glutamate activity can be neurotoxic and is implicated in conditions such as epilepsy, Alzheimer's disease, and neurodegenerative disorders. Imbalances in glutamate are also associated with mood disorders like depression and bipolar disorder.

Endorphins – These neuropeptides act as natural painkillers and mood enhancers, reducing stress and increasing pleasure. They are released during activities such as exercise (the "runner's high"), laughter, and social bonding.

Acetylcholine (ACh) – Plays a key role in attention, learning, memory, and muscle movement. While its direct influence on mood is less studied, imbalances can affect cognitive function and emotional stability. A decline in acetylcholine is associated with neurodegenerative conditions like Alzheimer's disease. It also plays a role in REM sleep regulation.

Oxytocin – Known as the "love hormone," oxytocin is crucial for bonding, trust, and social interactions. It reduces stress, promotes emotional connections, and enhances empathy. However, it also has a complex role in social behavior, as it may increase in-group favoritism and decrease trust toward outsiders.

Histamine – Though primarily known for its role in immune response and allergic reactions, histamine also acts as a neurotransmitter that regulates wakefulness, attention, and arousal.

It plays a role in mood and cognitive function, with disruptions linked to conditions such as schizophrenia and sleep disorders.

Related Hormone: Cortisol While cortisol is not classified as a neurotransmitter, it is a stress hormone that plays a crucial role in influencing mood by interacting with serotonin, dopamine, norepinephrine, and GABA. Secreted by the adrenal glands in response to stress, cortisol regulates metabolism, immune function, and blood sugar levels. However, chronic elevation of cortisol levels can contribute to anxiety, depression, and cognitive dysfunction, whereas reduced cortisol levels may result in fatigue and diminished motivation. Effective stress management through physical exercise, meditation, and adequate sleep is vital for maintaining balanced cortisol levels and overall mental health.

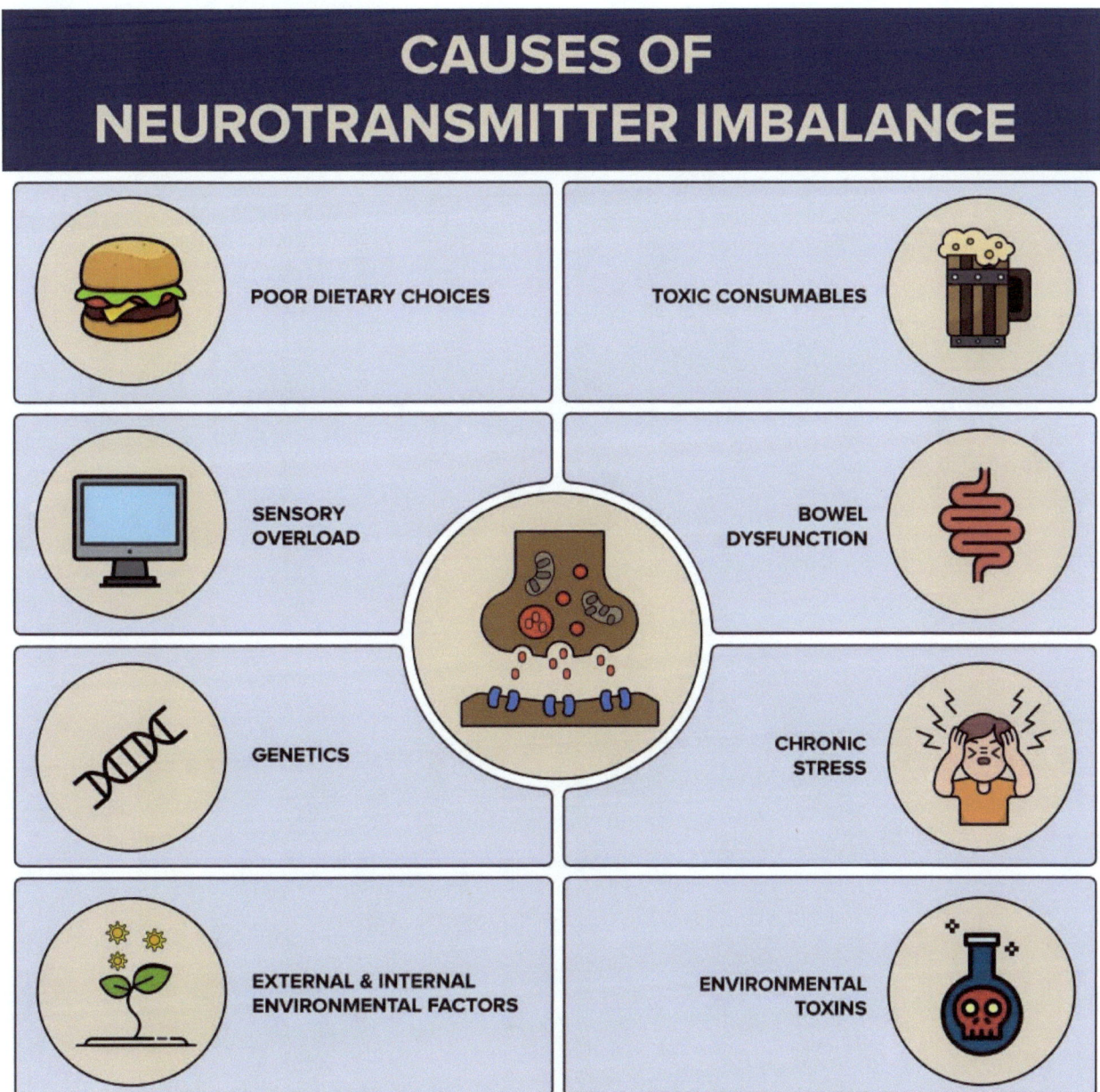

CAUSES OF NEUROTRANSMITTER IMBALANCE

POOR DIETARY CHOICES

TOXIC CONSUMABLES

SENSORY OVERLOAD

BOWEL DYSFUNCTION

GENETICS

CHRONIC STRESS

EXTERNAL & INTERNAL ENVIRONMENTAL FACTORS

ENVIRONMENTAL TOXINS

https://www.xcode.life/genes-and-health/what-neurotransmitter-causes-depression/

References:

Goodman & Gilman's: The Pharmacological Basis of Therapeutics, 13e. (2018). McGraw Hill Medical.
https://accessmedicine.mhmedical.com/content.aspx?bookid=2189§ionid=165936845&utm_source=chatgpt.com

Molecular Neuropharmacology: A Foundation for Clinical Neuroscience, 3E. (2015). McGraw Hill Medical.
https://accessbiomedicalscience.mhmedical.com/content.aspx?bookid=1204§ionid=72648538&utm_source=chatgpt.com

McEwen, B. S. (2007). Physiology and neurobiology of stress and adaptation: central role of the brain. Physiological Reviews, 87(3), 873–904.
https://doi.org/10.1152/physrev.00041.2006

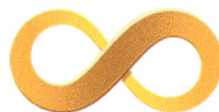

In a world saturated by screens, we've grown increasingly comfortable with fiction and disturbingly detached from reality. Hollywood and the broader entertainment industry have mastered the art of storytelling. But in doing so, they've also shaped belief systems, numbed emotional sensitivity, and altered the way people perceive violence, trauma, and even the value of life itself.

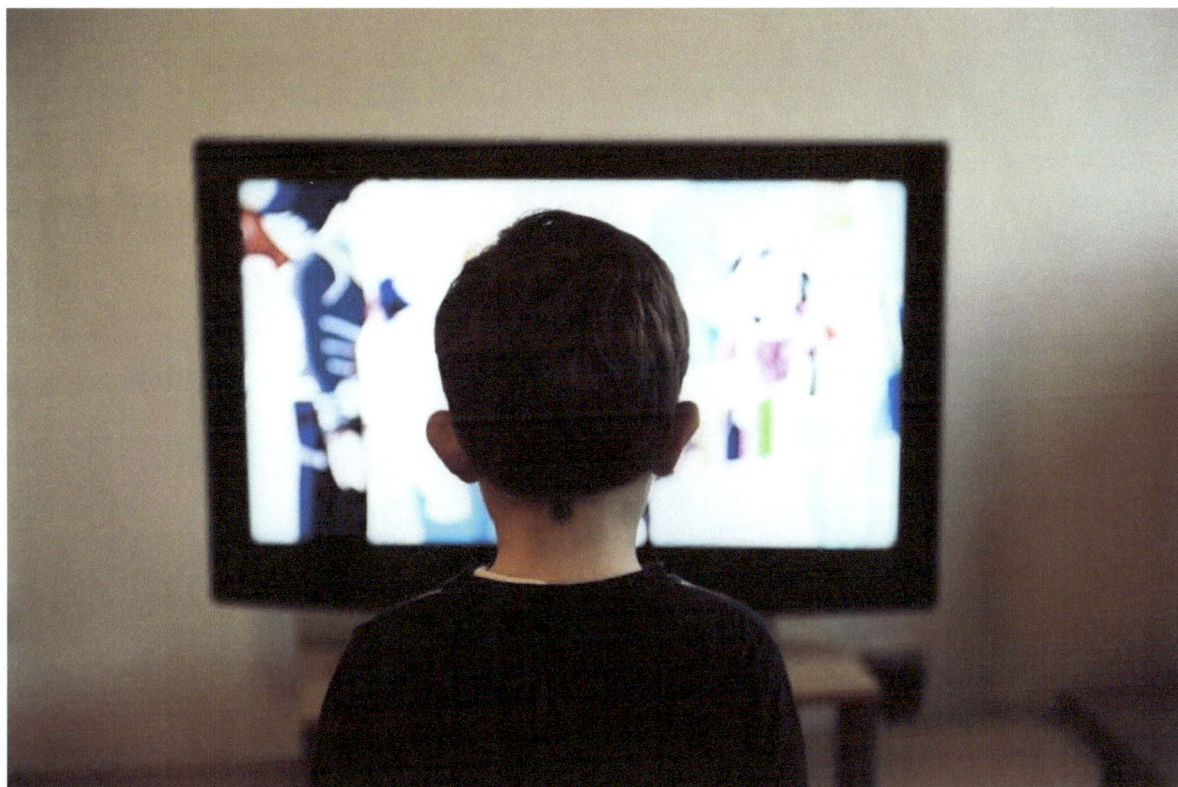

Television and film often depict firearms and violence with dramatic flair. Police officers re-holster their weapons carelessly, never checking to see if clothing or gear might catch the trigger, something that, in real life, could end in a tragic accident. Striker-fired firearms are shown making mechanical "cocking" sounds they don't make. Characters rack their slides as if they didn't already have a round chambered, an absurd notion in any tactical reality. These stylistic choices aren't just errors; they are illusions that condition audiences, especially those with no firsthand experience, to misunderstand basic truths about safety, readiness, and consequences. These aren't just cinematic tropes. They are forms of social psychological conditioning.

It doesn't stop at guns. In the world of TV and movies, violence is almost romanticized. Characters get shot multiple times and continue fighting as if pain and blood loss were minor inconveniences. Others are beaten senseless, only to rally with a defiant quip. No one suffers hearing damage from repeated gunfire in enclosed spaces. No one shows the tremors, the dissociation, or the collapse that often follows real trauma. Instead, they move on, undamaged, both physically and emotionally.

And therein lies one of the most disturbing consequences of modern media: **Desensitization**. We've reached a point where viewers can witness a character suffering what would be a fatal injury in real life and feel nothing. Not because they're cold-hearted, but because the medium has trained them not to feel. Life on screen resets with the next episode. A person shot or killed vanishes into the storyline with little more than a dramatic soundtrack and a fade to black.

But in real life, death doesn't come and go that easily. When someone dies, whether it's a law enforcement officer, a civilian, or even someone who committed a crime, a ripple effect spreads. Families grieve. Communities are shaken. Colleagues carry guilt and trauma. Witnesses replay events in their minds for years. The emotional, spiritual, and psychological consequences last long after the physical event has ended.

Hollywood doesn't show this. It rarely shows the tears of a mother, the PTSD of a survivor, the hollow silence in a family's home. It doesn't explore the real-life breakdowns, the isolation, or the long path of emotional recovery. And so, people lose touch, not just with how trauma actually works, but with the value of life itself.

This disconnection is one of the greatest threats to modern wellness. Because true wellness is not just physical, it's emotional, mental, and moral. It means feeling deeply. It means recognizing the weight of a life, even a fictional one. It means resisting the urge to become numb just because society finds comfort in distraction.

We are witnessing a cultural side effect of prolonged exposure to stylized violence: a loss of reverence for human life. It's not enough to simply say "it's just entertainment." When entertainment becomes education, as it so often does, we must question what we are being taught. And what we are unconsciously absorbing. This is where social psychology and holistic wellness intersect. We are not just bodies reacting to the world. We are minds and hearts shaped by it. When the culture around us numbs our response to suffering, we lose our connection to empathy, discernment, and truth.

Holistic health isn't just about food, exercise, or stress. It's about awareness. Emotional, mental, spiritual. It's the ability to stay awake in a world that lulls us to sleep through entertainment. It's seeing through the illusion, and reclaiming our human response to life, death, and everything in between.

So let's start noticing what we're being shown. Let's teach our young people that not everything on screen is real or right. Let's cultivate empathy, emotional intelligence, and the courage to feel deeply in a culture that tells us to feel nothing.

We must reconnect as holistic practitioners, wellness seekers, and aware human beings. We must pull back from the illusion and sit in the truth: trauma is not glamorous. Violence is not clean. Death, no matter whose it is, is not an empty plot device.

So, let's start by protecting not just our bodies, but our minds and hearts. Let's choose awareness over apathy, and discernment over blind acceptance. Let's challenge the stories we're fed and hold space for the reality they often ignore. Because if we don't, we risk becoming a society that feels nothing when life is lost. And that, more than any special effect, is the real tragedy.

The Effects of Viewing Media Violence

Learning Objective Question: What is the violence-viewing effect?

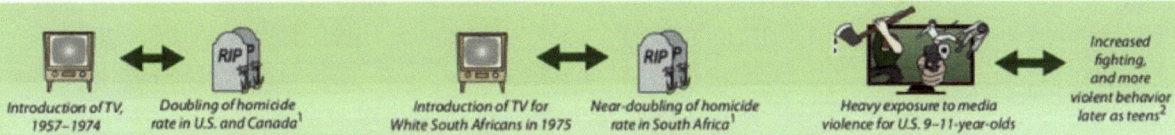

Introduction of TV, 1957–1974 ↔ Doubling of homicide rate in U.S. and Canada[1]	Introduction of TV for White South Africans in 1975 ↔ Near-doubling of homicide rate in South Africa[1]	Heavy exposure to media violence for U.S. 9–11-year-olds ↔ Increased fighting, and more violent behavior later as teens[2]

BUT, CORRELATION ≠ CAUSATION!

Experimental studies have also found that media violence viewing can **cause** aggression:

Viewing violence (compared to entertaining nonviolence) ➜ participants react more cruelly when provoked. (Effect is strongest if the violent person is attractive, the violence seems justified and realistic, the act goes unpunished, and the viewer does not see pain or harm caused.)

What prompts the *violence-viewing effect*?

1 IMITATION:

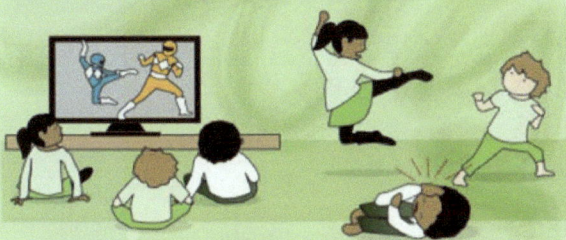

Watching violent cartoons ➜ Sevenfold increase in violent play[3]

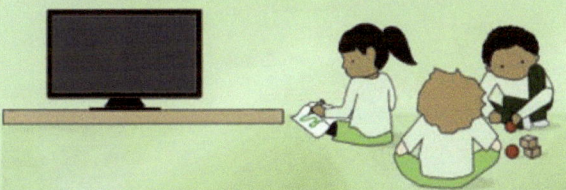

Limited exposure to violent programs ➜ Reduced aggressive behavior[4]

2 DESENSITIZATION:

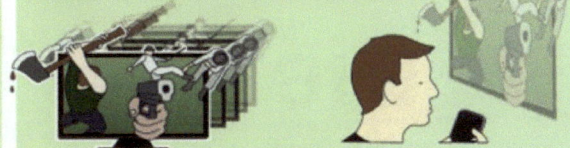

Prolonged exposure to violence ➜ Viewers are later indifferent (desensitized) to violence on TV or in real life.[5]

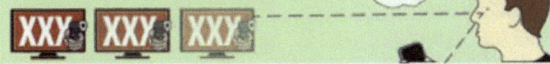

meh

Adult males spent 3 evenings watching sexually violent movies. ➜ Viewers became progressively less bothered by the violence shown. Compared to a control group, they expressed less sympathy for domestic violence victims and rated victims' injuries as less severe.[6]

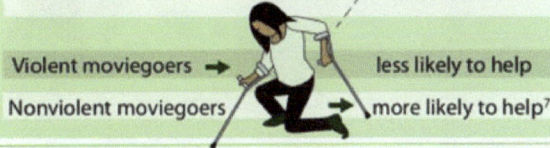

Violent moviegoers ➜ less likely to help

Nonviolent moviegoers ➜ more likely to help[7]

• **APA Task Force on Violent Media (2015)** found that the "research demonstrates a consistent relation between violent video game use and increases in aggressive behavior, aggressive cognitions, and aggressive affect, and decreases in prosocial behavior, empathy, and sensitivity to aggression."

• **American Academy of Pediatrics (2009)** has advised pediatricians that "media violence can contribute to aggressive behavior, desensitization to violence, nightmares, and fear of being harmed."

1. Centerwall, 1989. 2. Boxer at al., 2009; Gentile et al., 2011; Gentile & Bushman, 2012. 3. Boyatzis et al., 1995. 4. Christakis et al., 2013. 5. Fanti et al., 2009; Rule & Ferguson, 1986. 6. Mullin & Linz, 1995. 7. Bushman & Anderson, 2009.

"Born With Nothing, Die With Nothing"

The concept of **"born with nothing, die with nothing"** is a profound philosophical idea found in many Eastern traditions, including Buddhism and Taoism. It reflects the principles of impermanence, detachment, and the cyclical nature of existence. We enter this world with no possessions, and when we leave, we take nothing with us. This underscores the transient nature of material wealth and highlights the deeper value of experiences, relationships, and inner growth.

Happiness is not about collecting material things or beautiful memories. It is about having a deep feeling of contentment and knowing that life is a blessing. – Jeigh Ilano

This idea extends beyond human life to all living beings, aligning with the concept of "no beginning, no end." Like the yin-yang (☯) and infinity (∞) symbols, it represents the continuous flow of transformation, where emptiness gives rise to form, and form dissolves back into emptiness.

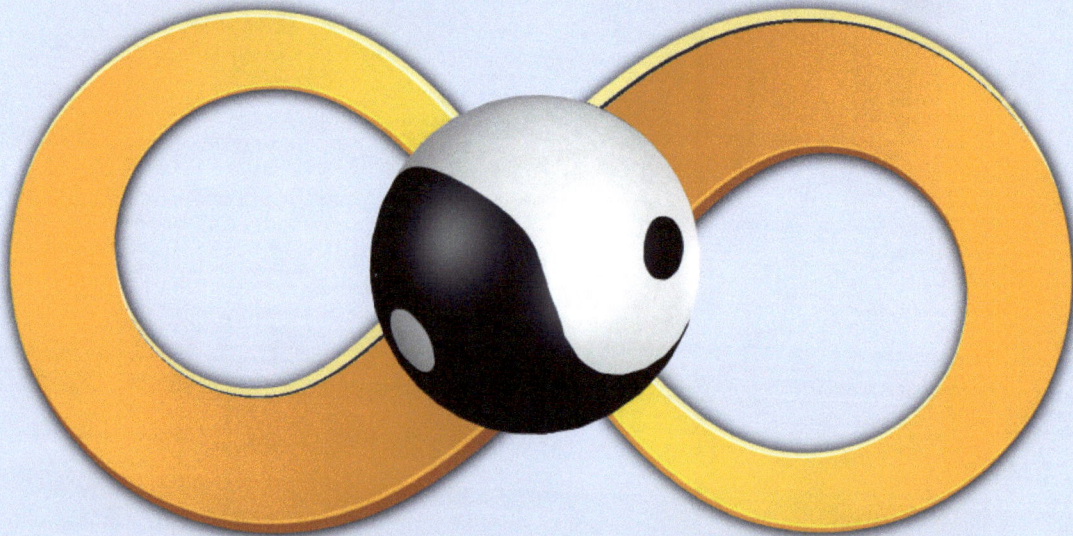

Born with Nothing, Die with Nothing

"Born with nothing, die with nothing" reflects the cyclical nature of existence not just humans but all living organisms, aligning with the concept of "no beginning, no end." Like the yin-yang and infinity symbols, it represents the continuous flow of transformation where emptiness gives rise to form, and form dissolving back into emptiness.

www.MindAndBodyExercises.com

© Copyright 2025 - CAD Graphics, Inc.

Human life can be seen as consciousness temporarily residing in form, experiencing the ever-shifting balance of existence before returning to the formless. In Taoism, this mirrors the **Dao (道)**, the ever-flowing source from which all things arise and to which they ultimately return. Just as yin transforms into yang and vice versa, life and death are not endpoints but expressions of an eternal process. This perspective encourages non-attachment, balance, and harmony with the natural flow of life, recognizing that all physical possessions are ultimately borrowed, and everything returns to the Dao.

Related Concepts:

Biblical Perspective: A similar idea appears in the Book of Job, where Job states, "The Lord gave, and the Lord has taken away; may the name of the Lord be praised." This is often interpreted as an acceptance of life's impermanence, acknowledging that all we have is ultimately a gift and can be withdrawn at any time.

The Heart Sutra: A central text in Mahayana Buddhism, the Heart Sutra articulates the nature of emptiness, stating that all phenomena bear the mark of emptiness—their true nature is beyond birth and death, being and non-being.

Śūnyatā (Emptiness): In Mahayana Buddhism, śūnyatā refers to the understanding that all things are devoid of intrinsic existence. This insight is fundamental to recognizing the transient nature of life and the absence of a permanent self.

Samsara: This term describes the continuous cycle of birth, death, and rebirth, emphasizing the impermanence and suffering inherent in worldly existence.

Why This Concept Matters in Everyday Life

Understanding and embracing this concept can have a profound impact on how we approach daily life. It reminds us to focus on what truly matters. Our experiences, relationships, and inner development are most important, rather than being overly attached to material possessions or fleeting successes. By recognizing the impermanent nature of all things, we can cultivate greater resilience and gratitude in the face of challenges, reduce unnecessary stress, and live with greater appreciation and mindfulness.

This perspective encourages us to be present in each moment, to value the people around us, and to engage in life with a sense of peace and acceptance. It also promotes generosity and compassion, as we recognize that nothing truly belongs to us, and what we give to others is ultimately part of the greater flow of all existence.
By implementing this understanding into our lives, we can develop a deeper sense of harmony, balance, and contentment, freeing ourselves from the burdens of attachment and fear while embracing the natural rhythms of life.

The Chinese character for humility is 谦 (qiān). The character for a king (or ruler) is 王 (wáng), but when flipped, it can be associated with something reversed, such as a reversed position, or lack of power. Combining these, one could interpret 谦王 (qiān wáng) as "humble ruler" or "modest king", representing a ruler who is both powerful and humble.

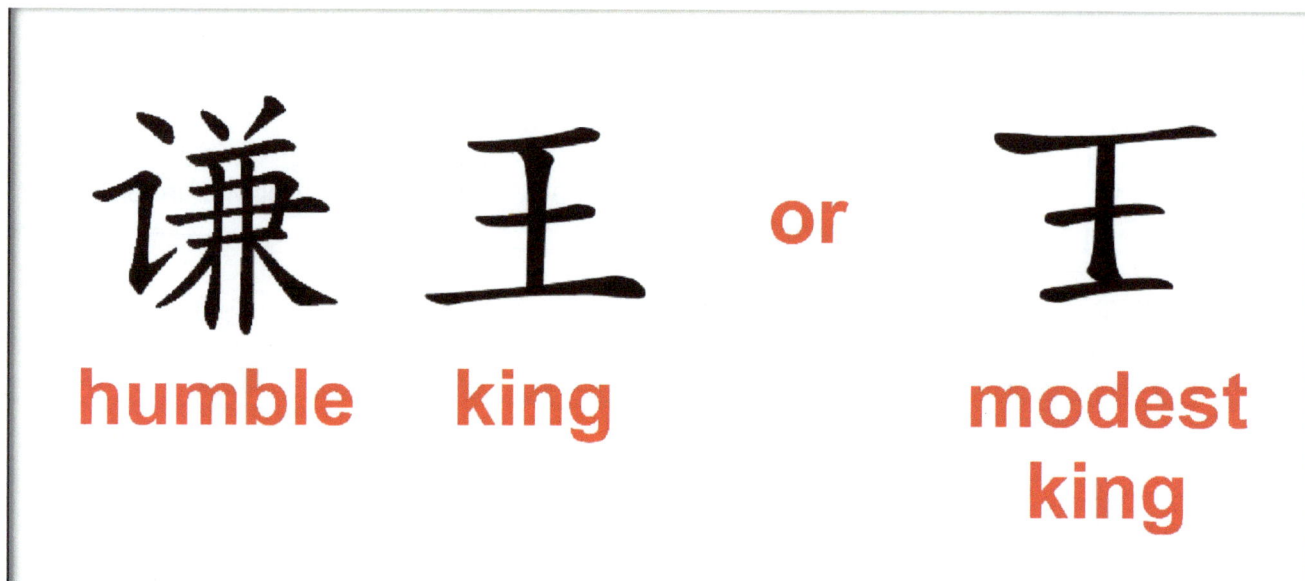

In a time long ago, a great king ruled over a vast and prosperous land. Despite his power, he felt something was missing. Perhaps an imbalance in the heart of his kingdom and perhaps within himself. Recognizing the limits of his own understanding, the king invited a wise man to help restore harmony to his realm.

The wise man accepted the invitation, bringing with him not armies or gold, but clarity, insight, and timeless wisdom. Through thoughtful guidance, he realigned the kingdom's priorities. Not by conquering enemies, but by restoring balance between the people and their values. He offered no lectures on dominance or strategy, but instead taught the king to listen more, act less, and lead from within. And then, without asking for any reward or recognition, the wise man quietly departed.

The king was stunned. He had expected a request for treasure or title. Instead, the king was left with only the echo of wisdom that had shifted the foundation of his being. He was no longer the same man. In honor of this transformative experience, the king ordered the Chinese character for "king" (王) to be turned upside down wherever it appeared in his palace.

This symbolic act was not a rejection of power, but rather a redefinition of it. By inverting the symbol of his own authority, the king declared a new truth:

Wisdom is greater than power. Humility is the highest throne.

The Deeper Meaning

While the tale may not be part of the classic canon of Chinese folklore, its message is deeply rooted in Eastern philosophy and holistic wisdom traditions.

In **Taoist** thought, the greatest rulers are often those who lead without force. The sage governs by aligning with the *Tao* or natural order, practicing *wu wei* or effortless action, and allowing things to unfold organically.

In **Confucian** ethics, the moral character of the ruler sets the tone for the nation. A wise and virtuous leader brings peace not through decrees but by embodying righteousness.

In **Buddhist** teachings, detachment from ego and recognition of impermanence guide the wise. Like the sage in the story, the Bodhisattva acts for the benefit of others without seeking personal gain.

The upside-down character becomes a living reminder: true power lies not in domination, but in service, awareness, and the willingness to learn.

A Reflection for Our Times

In today's world, where leadership is often equated with control, and success with status, the *Upside-Down King* offers us a timeless teaching:

Sometimes, the greatest transformation comes not from gaining more, but from surrendering pride and embracing wisdom.

This story reminds us that holistic well-being begins with humility, whether we are leading others, caring for our health, or walking the path of self-discovery. The body may follow orders, but the soul responds to truth. And in the realm of wellness, just as in the kingdom of the wise king, balance is restored when wisdom reigns over ego.

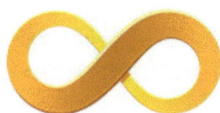

"Heaven and Earth, Turned Upside Down"

"Heaven and Earth, Turned Upside Down" is a phrase that means a complete and radical upheaval or change, signifying a situation where the established order is completely disrupted and everything is thrown into chaos as if the natural order of the universe has been reversed; essentially, a dramatic and significant change where the normal way of things is completely overturned.

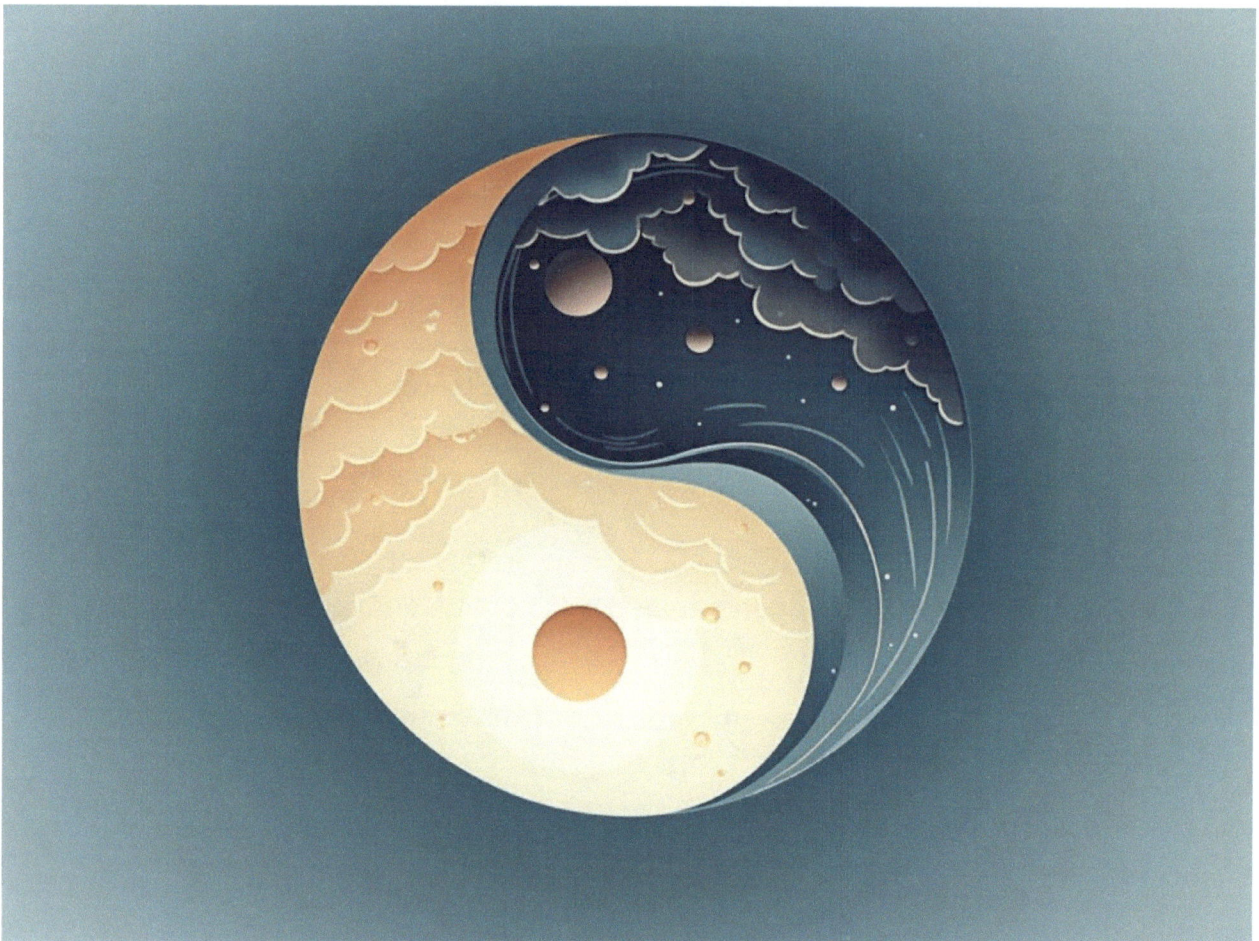

The concept of "Heaven and Earth, turned upside down" appears in various Chinese philosophical and esoteric traditions, including Daoism (I Ching), and martial arts. It often symbolizes a reversal of natural order, transformation, or a shift in perception.

Possible Interpretations:

1. **Reversal of Cosmic Order**

- o Normally, Heaven (Yang) is above, and Earth (Yin) is below. Flipping this order suggests a paradox, disorder, or a fundamental transformation of reality.

- o It can imply chaos, breaking norms, or a cosmic shift that forces new perspectives.

2. **Daoist Alchemy & Inner Transformation**

- o In Daoist internal alchemy (Neidan), reversing Heaven and Earth can symbolize inner transformation, where the ordinary world is transcended.

- o It is sometimes associated with the *Microcosmic Orbit* practice, where energy (*Qi*) circulates against its usual flow to achieve spiritual enlightenment.

3. **I Ching Influence**

- o Certain hexagrams in the I Ching hint at the reversal of Heaven and Earth, representing a dramatic change, like Hexagram 12 (Pí, Stagnation) vs. Hexagram 11 (Tài, Peace).

- o When the natural order is disrupted, it can indicate a need for adaptation, renewal, or a deeper understanding of balance.

4. **Martial Arts & Strategy**

- o Some martial philosophies refer to this idea in unexpected tactics, adaptability, and overturning conventional wisdom in combat.

- o It relates to Sun Tzu's "Art of War" principles, where flipping the expected order creates strategic advantage.

5. **Spiritual Awakening & Perception Shift**

- o A mystical interpretation suggests seeing beyond illusion *(Maya)* or breaking free from conventional thought.

- o It resonates with Zen and Chan Buddhism's use of paradox to awaken deeper understanding.

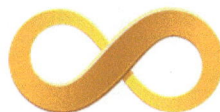

119

SECTION V: Spiritual Wisdom & Philosophical Reflections

The Eight Keys of Wisdom

The **Eight Keys of Wisdom** are rooted in **Taoist, Confucian, and Buddhist principles**, such as:

- **Wu Wei (Effortless Action)** in Taoism, similar to "Be Like Bamboo" (flexibility and balance).

- **Right Conduct and Ethics** in Confucianism, similar to "The True-Right-Correct Method."

- **Mindfulness and Detachment from Thought** in Buddhism are reflected in "Stop Being Drunk on Your Own Thoughts."

Eight Keys of Wisdom

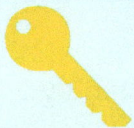 **Reflection**

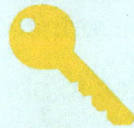 **Attain honor**

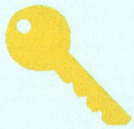 **Make correct choices**

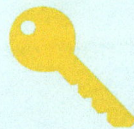 **Change your reality**

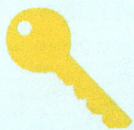 **Overcome your delusion**

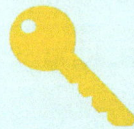 **Become a vessel of wisdom**

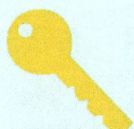 **Turn on your light**

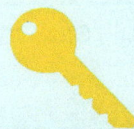 **Draw from nature's energies**

www.MindAndBodyExercises.com

© Copyright 2025 - CAD Graphics, Inc.

The **Eight Keys of Wisdom** serve as guiding principles for integrating mindfulness and meditation into daily life. Here's a deeper look at each:

1. Reflection (Know Your True Self)
- This key emphasizes self-awareness and authenticity.

- It encourages recognizing personal strengths, weaknesses, and emotional patterns.

- Understanding oneself allows for conscious decision-making and alignment with one's true nature.

2. Make Correct Choices (The True-Right-Correct Method)
- Rooted in Eastern philosophy, this principle teaches the importance of seeking truth and making ethical choices.

- "True" represents inner wisdom, "Right" signifies ethical action, and "Correct" ensures that actions align with both personal integrity and universal balance.

3. Overcome Delusion (Stop Being Drunk on Your Own Thoughts)
- Encourages detachment from overthinking and emotional reactivity.

- Teaches mindfulness techniques to observe thoughts without being consumed by them.

- Helps develop clarity and inner calm by breaking free from habitual negative thinking.

4. How Will You Be Remembered? (Plant Good Seeds)
- Invites reflection on one's legacy and the impact of actions on others.

- Encourages living with purpose, kindness, and awareness of how one's presence affects the world.

- Turn on your light, becoming an inspiration and not a warning to others

5. Seek Connectedness & Honor (Be Like a Mountain)
- Focuses on building meaningful relationships through respect, integrity, and compassion.

- Recognizes the interconnectedness of all people and the importance of honoring those connections.

- Teaches that true strength comes from unity rather than isolation.

6. Change Your Reality for the Better
- Encourages personal responsibility in shaping one's experiences.

- Highlights the power of perspective—choosing optimism and proactive behavior over victimhood.

- Teaches how shifting internal attitudes can influence external circumstances.

7. Become a Vessel of Wisdom (It Only Takes One Match to Light a Thousand)
- Demonstrates the power of small actions in creating widespread change.

- Encourages leading by example, where one positive act can inspire many others.

- Stresses that transformation begins with individual effort, no matter how small.

8. Draw from Nature's Energies (Be Like Bamboo)
- Symbolizes resilience, flexibility, and strength.

- Encourages adaptability in the face of challenges while maintaining inner strength.

- Teaches that true power lies in balance, being strong yet flexible, firm yet yielding.

The **Eight Keys of Wisdom** are rooted in **Taoist, Confucian, and Buddhist principles**, such as:

- **Wu Wei (Effortless Action)** in Taoism, similar to "Be Like Bamboo" (flexibility and balance).

- **Right Conduct and Ethics** in Confucianism, similar to "The True-Right-Correct Method."

- **Mindfulness and Detachment from Thought** in Buddhism are reflected in "Stop Being Drunk on Your Own Thoughts."

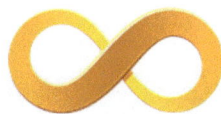

*The **Eightfold Path*** in Buddhism and the ***Eight Keys of Wisdom*** both emphasize self-awareness, ethical living, and inner transformation, but they approach wisdom from different angles. Buddhism focuses on liberation from suffering and Taoism emphasizes harmony with the *Tao* (the Way). Below are summaries and correlations between them.

The Eightfold Path
Right Livelihood

Right Speech · Right View · Right Action · Right Effort · Right Mindfulness · Right Concentration · Right Intention

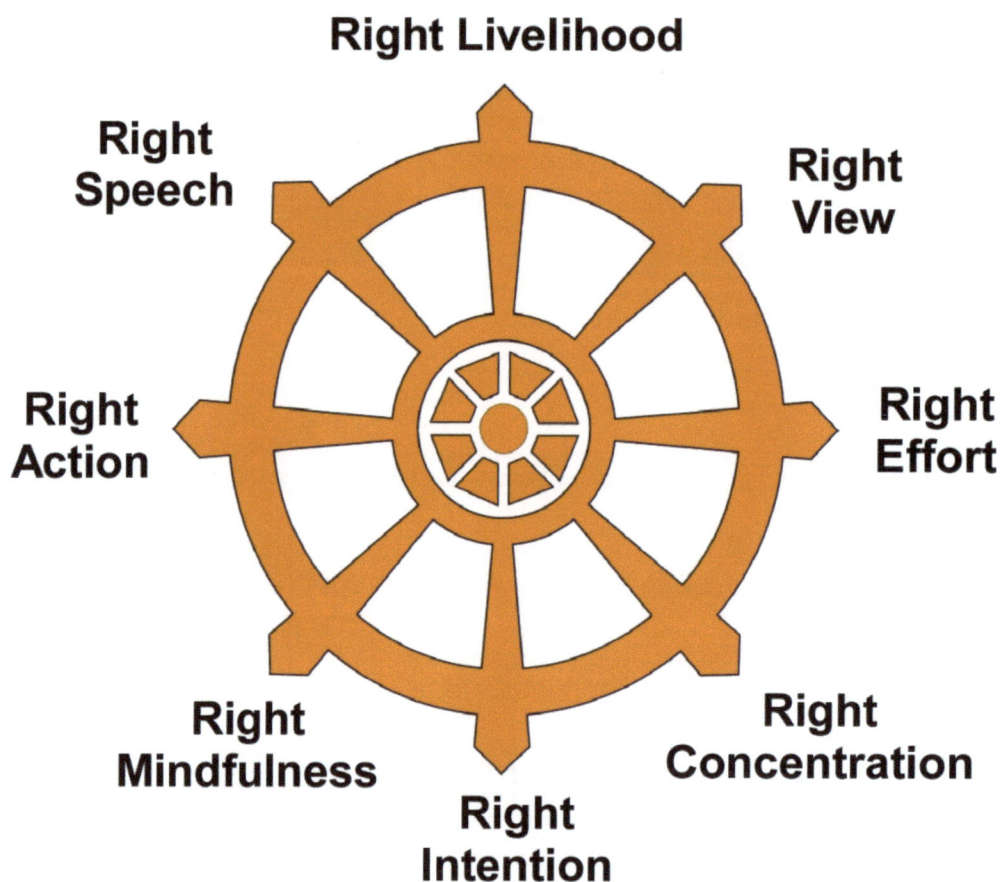

The **Buddhist Eightfold Path** is a core teaching of the Buddha, forming the practical aspect of the *Four Noble Truths*. It guides ethical conduct, mental discipline, and wisdom, leading to the cessation of suffering and enlightenment (*nirvana*).

The Eightfold Path consists of:

Wisdom (Prajñā / Panna)

1. **Right View (Sammā-diṭṭhi)** – Understanding the Four Noble Truths and seeing reality as it is.

2. **Right Intention (Sammā-saṅkappa)** – Cultivating thoughts of goodwill, and harmlessness, avoiding harmful desires and ill-will.

Ethical Conduct (Śīla / Sīla)

3. **Right Speech (Sammā-vācā)** – Speaking truthfully, kindly, and avoiding lying, gossip, or harmful words

4. **Right Action (Sammā-kammanta)** – Acting ethically by resisting from harming living beings, stealing, and engaging in improper sexual conduct.

5. **Right Livelihood (Sammā-ājīva)** – Earning a living in a way that does not cause harm or exploit others.

Mental Discipline (Samādhi)

6. **Right Effort (Sammā-vāyāma)** – Cultivating positive states of mind, preventing negative thoughts, and striving for self-improvement.

7. **Right Mindfulness (Sammā-sati)** – Maintaining awareness of one's body, feelings, thoughts, and phenomena through consistent mindfulness practice.

8. **Right Concentration (Sammā-samādhi)** – Developing deep meditative states of focus to achieve insight and tranquility.

Like the Eightfold Path, The Eight Keys of Wisdom is a core teaching in ancient wisdom, drawing from Taoism, Buddhism, and Confucianism. It guides ethical conduct, mental discipline, and wisdom, leading to the cessation of suffering and enlightenment (*nirvana*).

Eight Keys of Wisdom

1. **Reflection** – See yourself as others see you

2. **Make correct choices** (Hun & Po) – Discerning true, right, and correct. Dealing with the inner conflict

3. **Overcome your delusion** – 5 agents, 7 distractions

4. **Turn on your light** – See and be seen, plant good seeds

5. **Be the mountain** – Attain honor rooted in principle

6. **Change your reality** – Assume responsibility of your fate or destiny

7. **Become a vessel of wisdom** – Practice what you preach, become a role model rather than a warning

8. **Water over fire** – Draw from nature's energies

Correlations Between the Eightfold Path and 8 Keys of Wisdom

1. **Reflection – Right View (Sammā-diṭṭhi)**

   o **Taoist Wisdom:** See yourself as others see you.

   o **Buddhist Parallel:** The Right View teaches seeing reality as it is, free from illusion. In Buddhism, self-awareness includes understanding how others perceive us and recognizing our attachments and biases.

2. **True, Right and Correct (Hun & Po) – Right Intention (Sammā-saṅkappa)**

   o **Taoist Wisdom:** Manage and cope with inner conflicts.

   o **Buddhist Parallel:** Right Intention involves aligning thoughts with ethical and wholesome goals, reducing inner conflict between desire (Po) and higher wisdom (Hun). Both traditions emphasize balancing these opposing aspects of the psyche.

3. **Overcome Your Delusion – Right Effort (Sammā-vāyāma)**

   o **Taoist Wisdom:** 5 agents, 7 distractions (Five Elements & Emotional Imbalances).

   o **Buddhist Parallel:** Right Effort means actively working to remove unwholesome states (such as greed, anger, and delusion) and cultivate wisdom. In Taoism, recognizing the interplay of the Five Elements and overcoming distractions aligns with maintaining mental clarity.

4. **Turn on Your Light – Right Mindfulness (Sammā-sati)**

- ○ **Taoist Wisdom:** See and be seen. Plant good seeds to leave a legacy of knowledge.

- ○ **Buddhist Parallel:** Right Mindfulness is about clear awareness of one's actions, emotions, and thoughts. "Turning on the light" in Taoism refers to conscious self-awareness, which aligns with the Buddhist practice of mindfulness meditation.

5. **Be the Mountain – Right Action (Sammā-kammanta)**

- ○ **Taoist Wisdom:** Achieve honor and respect by being rooted in principle.

- ○ **Buddhist Parallel:** Right Action means living with integrity, abstaining from harm and unethical behavior. Being "the mountain" represents stability in virtue, just as Right Action is about unwavering moral conduct.

6. **Change Your Reality – Right Livelihood (Sammā-ājīva)**

- ○ **Taoist Wisdom:** Assume responsibility for your fate or destiny.

- ○ **Buddhist Parallel:** Right Livelihood encourages earning a living ethically and shaping one's future through right choices. Taoism's view that we shape our destiny aligns with Buddhism's emphasis on karma and responsibility for one's path.

7. **Become the Vessel of Wisdom – Right Speech (Sammā-vācā)**

- ○ **Taoist Wisdom:** Practice what you preach. Strive to live as an example and not a warning to others.

- ○ **Buddhist Parallel:** Right Speech teaches honest, compassionate communication. In Taoism, becoming a "vessel of wisdom" means embodying truth, much like Right Speech requires sincerity in words.

8. **Water Over Fire – Right Concentration (Sammā-samādhi)**

- ○ **Taoist Wisdom:** Balance the elements; maintain peace in chaos.

- ○ **Buddhist Parallel:** Right Concentration cultivates mental stillness and deep meditative absorption, similar to Taoist teachings on harmonizing the forces of water (yin) and fire (yang) to maintain balance and clarity.

The 8-Step Path to Achieve the Best Version of You

A long-understood method of achieving harmony between one's mind, body and spirit, is this 8-Step Path. It has its origin in the ancient Chinese philosophy of Daoism but is highly relative to modern culture. The figure "8" is important to understand that as the infinity circle, there is no beginning nor end to entering into this process. It is a journey of self-awareness that can be entered into at any point throughout one's lifetime. Life is a challenge, and so is staying on this path of self-improvement. The reward is at the end of one's journey, knowing that they have pursued a meaningful life with direction and purpose.

1 Learning to Know Your "True Self"

By seeing & understanding your nature, self-reflection opens the door to the other steps of this process.

2 Making Correct Daily Choices

True

Right — Correct

Awareness of an inner "Moral Compass" to balance decisions by understanding true, right & correct.

3 Overcome Delusion of Your Thoughts & Ideas

You are not your thoughts. As consciousness you control your thoughts. Try not to be swayed by the mundane & trivial. Be solid like the root & not flippant like the leaves.

4 Cultivate Good Seeds to Pass On

Realize that you have a higher purpose beyond gaining material wealth and status. Be the light at the end of the tunnel.

5 Attain Honor

Live by principle - stand firm in what you believe, while allowing challenges to flow around you. Stand like a mountain, flow like a river.

6 Change Your Reality

Understand that you are in control of your life and the choices you make determine your success or failure within your reality.

7 Become a Living Vessel of Wisdom

Knowledge alone is not power. The sharing of our knowledge is when knowledge becomes powerful.

8 Draw on Nature's Power

Qigong   Tai Chi   Baguazhang

Cultivate a strong mind, body & spirit by connecting to nature's fire, water & wind with sitting, standing & moving exercises.

128

© Copyright 2018 – CAO Graphics, Inc

Buddhist Eightfold Path	Taoist Eight Keys of Wisdom	Core Similarity
Right View (Sammā-diṭṭhi)	Reflection – See yourself as others see you	Self-awareness & perceiving reality as it is
Right Intention (Sammā-saṅkappa)	Po & Hun – Deal with the inner conflict	Aligning thoughts with wisdom and balance
Right Effort (Sammā-vāyāma)	Overcome Your Delusion – 5 agents, 7 distractions	Removing distractions & cultivating clarity
Right Mindfulness (Sammā-sati)	Turn on Your Light – See and be seen	Awareness of self and surroundings
Right Action (Sammā-kammanta)	Be the Mountain – Rooted in principle	Stability in moral conduct
Right Livelihood (Sammā-ājīva)	Change Your Reality – Assume responsibility for your destiny	Ethical living & shaping one's future
Right Speech (Sammā-vācā)	Become the Vessel of Wisdom – Practice what you preach	Integrity in words & actions
Right Concentration (Sammā-samādhi)	Water Over Fire – Balance the elements	Mental stillness & harmonizing opposites

The phrase, *"True words are seldom kind. Kind words are seldom true,"* highlights the balance between truth and kindness, with correctness arising from their synthesis.

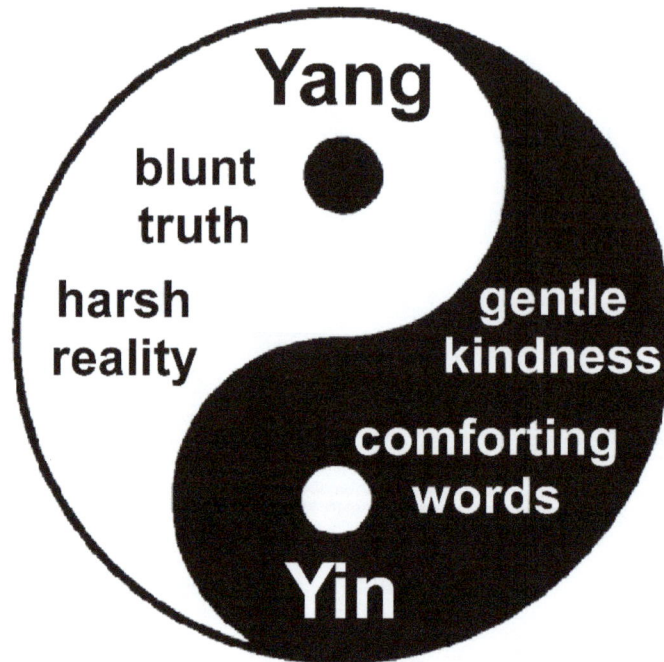

Yin and Yang in Truth and Kindness

- **Truth (Yang – Hard, Objective, Direct):** Truth is clear and straightforward, focusing on facts rather than perceptions. It aligns with the logical aspect of "rightness," emphasizing what is accurate over emotional considerations. Similar to yang, truth clarifies reality without prioritizing comfort.

- **Kindness (Yin – Soft, Subjective, Nurturing):** Kindness is based on empathy and the emotional aspect of interactions. It often aims to soften the impact of truth in order to maintain harmony and relationships. This relates to the emotional side of "truthfulness," focusing on how something feels rather than its factual accuracy. Similar to yin, kindness nurtures and soothes, sometimes prioritizing comfort over complete disclosure.

Correctness as the Balance

Neither extreme—blunt truth nor gentle avoidance—leads to effective communication. The optimal form of communication balances emotional sensitivity and logical correctness.

Wisdom involves knowing when to emphasize accuracy, when to offer empathy, and how to integrate both aspects.

Similar to how yin and yang transform under specific conditions, truth can be softened by kindness without compromising its integrity, while kindness can convey truth without becoming misleading. The skill of achieving balance lies in articulating what is true *appropriately,* ensuring it is both logically accurate and emotionally resonant.

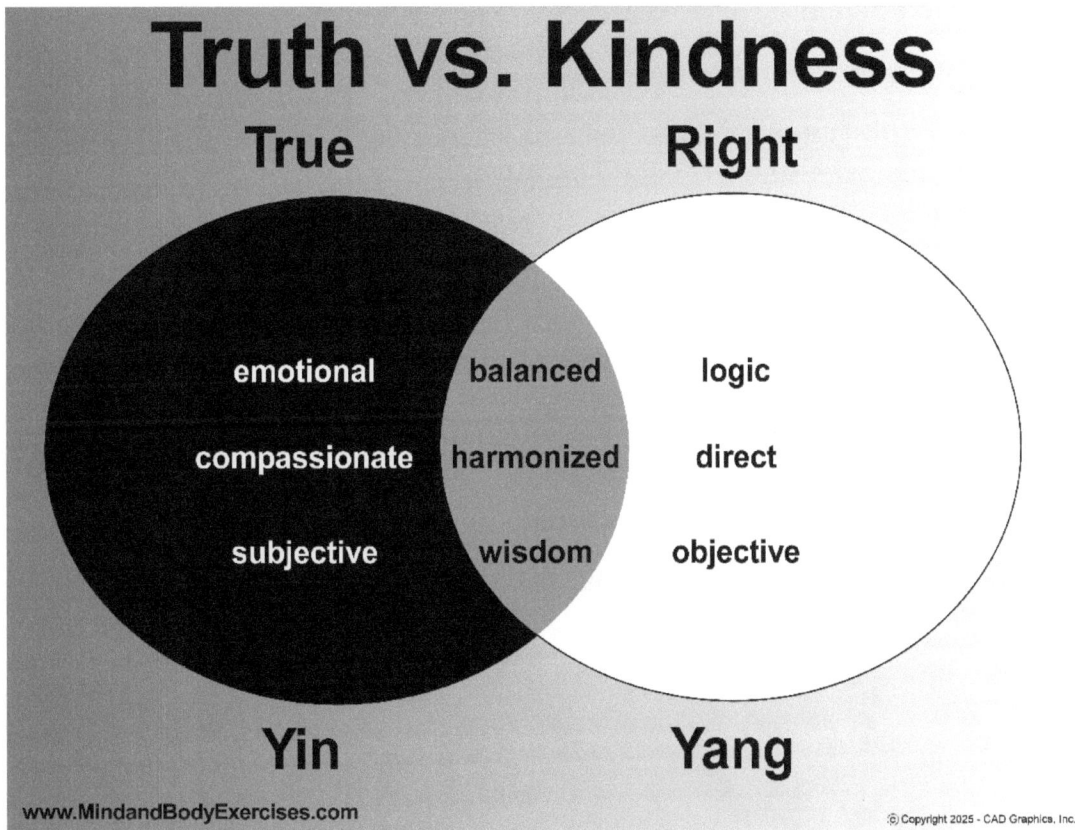

Truth vs. Kindness

True — Right

emotional | balanced | logic

compassionate | harmonized | direct

subjective | wisdom | objective

Yin — Yang

www.MindandBodyExercises.com

© Copyright 2025 - CAD Graphics, Inc.

Real-Life Examples of Truth vs. Kindness

1. **Health & Well-Being:**

   o **Pure Truth (Yang):** A doctor bluntly tells a patient, "You are dangerously overweight, and you need to lose weight immediately, or you risk serious health issues."

   o **Pure Kindness (Yin):** "You're perfect just the way you are. Don't worry about your weight."

   o **Balanced (Correct – Yin-Yang):** "Your health is important, and I want to support you in making changes that will help you feel better and live longer."

2. **Relationships & Personal Growth:**

- **Pure Truth (Yang):** A friend tells another, "Your behavior is selfish, and that's why people distance themselves from you."

- **Pure Kindness (Yin):** "You're wonderful just as you are. Everyone should accept you without question."

- **Balanced (Correct – Yin-Yang):** "I value you as a friend, and I've noticed that some of your actions push people away. Would you be open to talking about ways to strengthen your relationships?"

3. **Work & Professional Feedback:**

- **Pure Truth (Yang):** A boss tells an employee, "Your work is subpar, and you might not last here if you don't improve."

- **Pure Kindness (Yin):** "You're doing just fine, no worries!" (even when the work needs improvement).

- **Balanced (Correct – Yin-Yang):** "I see your potential, and I think with some focused effort in these areas, you could perform at a higher level. I'd love to help you get there."

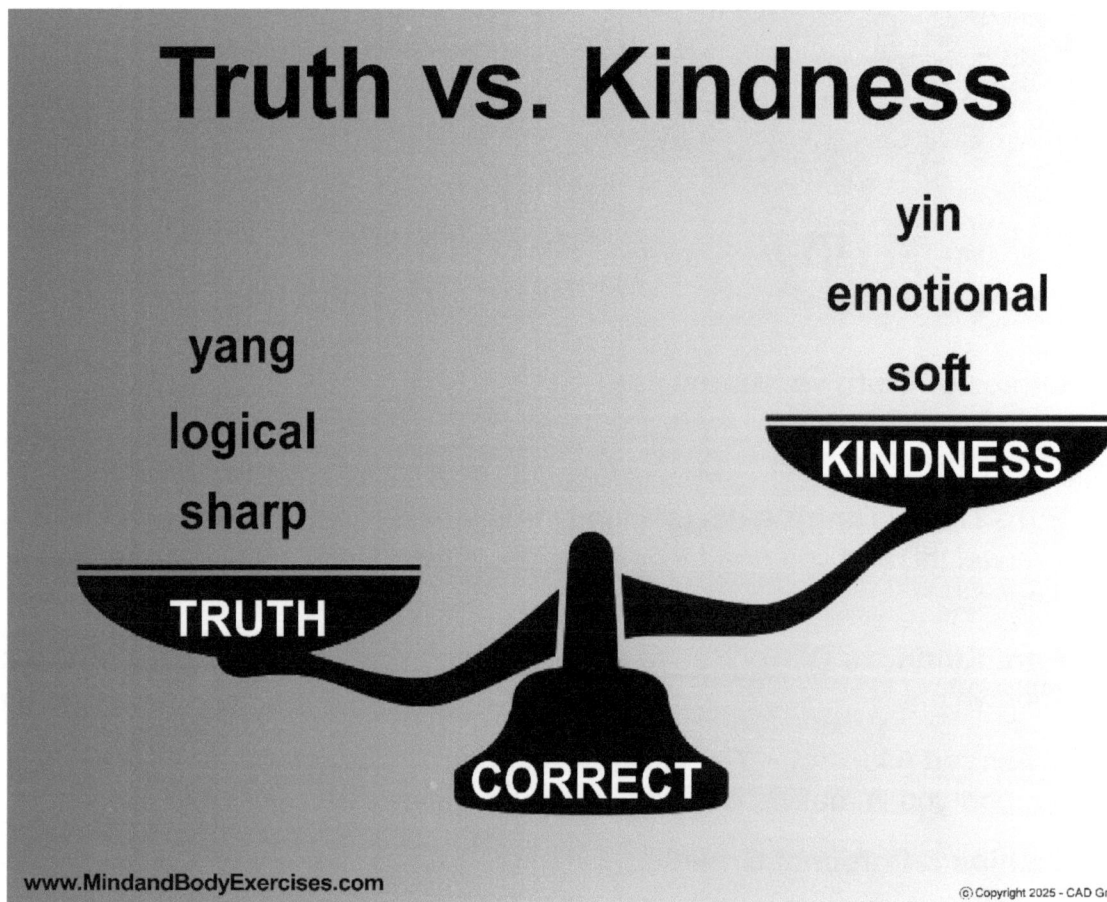

Truth vs. Kindness

yang
logical
sharp

TRUTH

yin
emotional
soft

KINDNESS

CORRECT

www.MindandBodyExercises.com

© Copyright 2025 - CAD Graphics, Inc.

"Man Divides Heaven and Earth"

The concept of **"Man divides Heaven and Earth"** is a fundamental idea in Chinese philosophy, particularly in Daoism and Confucian thought. It relates to the idea that humanity serves as a bridge between **Heaven (天, Tiān)** and **Earth (地, Dì)**—two fundamental cosmic forces.

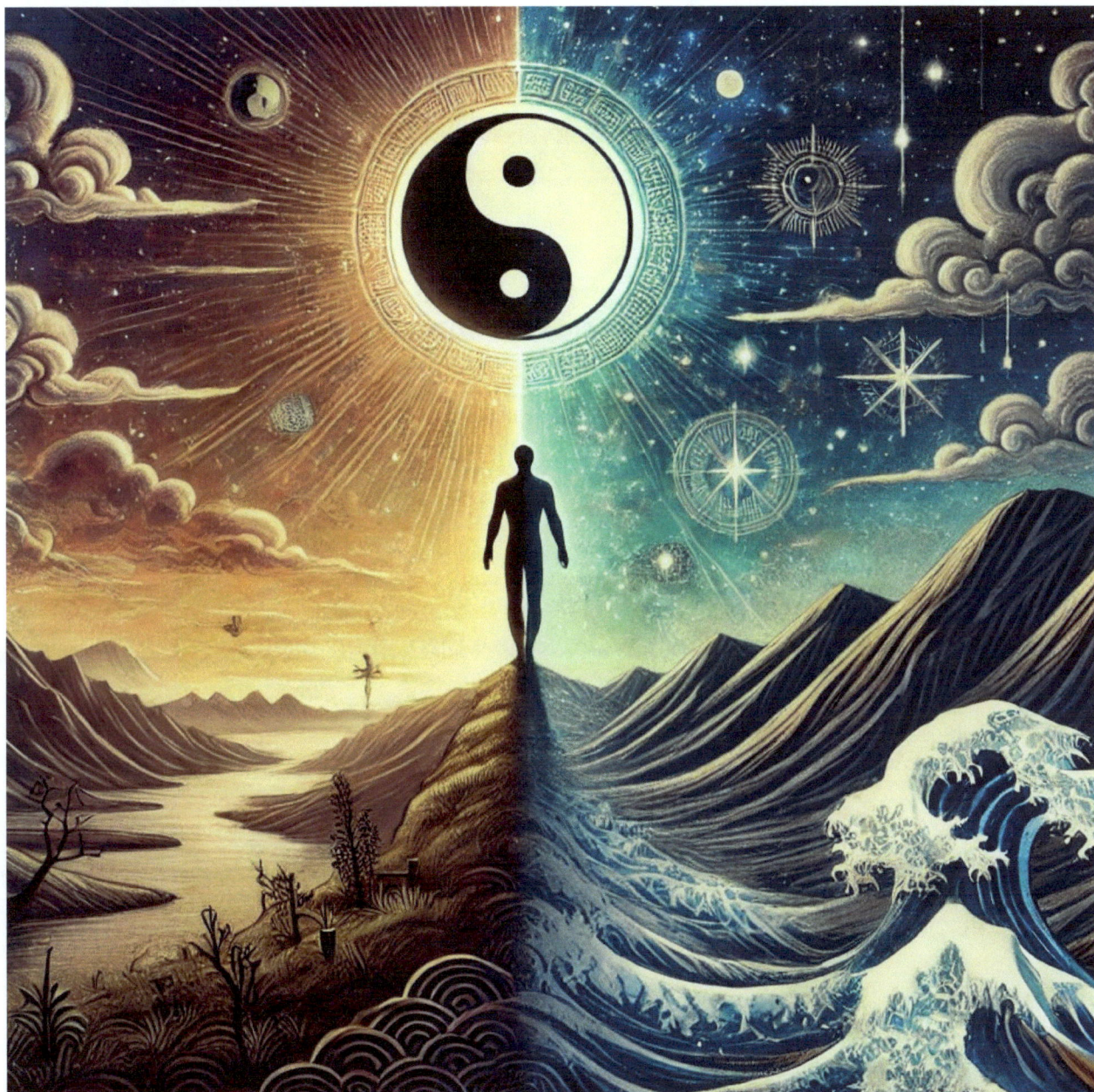

Key Aspects of the Concept:

1. **The Triad of Heaven, Earth, and Man**

   o Heaven represents the formless, the celestial, the spiritual, and the governing natural laws.

   o Earth represents the material, the manifested, the physical world, and stability.

   o Man is the mediator, possessing both spiritual (Heaven) and physical (Earth) aspects.

   o Humans impose order, create divisions, and establish structures to align with the Dao.

2. **Humanity as the Harmonizer**

   o Humans have the unique ability to observe natural rhythms (from Heaven) and adapt them to earthly existence.

   o Through philosophy, morality, and governance, humans bring order, such as dividing time into calendars, measuring space, and establishing social structures.

3. **Yin-Yang and Five Elements Influence**

   o This idea ties into yin-yang theory because man, in the middle, balances opposing forces.

   o It also aligns with the Five Elements (or Phases) (Wu Xing) since humans categorize and interact with nature based on these elemental relationships.

4. **Practical Applications**

   o In Confucianism, it applies to ethics, social roles, and proper conduct.

   o In Daoism, it relates to aligning human actions with the Dao and achieving balance.

   o In traditional Chinese medicine (TCM), it explains the body's role as a microcosm of the universe.

In today's evolving conversation around holistic health, enlightenment is resurfacing-not just as an esoteric ideal, but as a practical and deep personal milestone within the journey toward total well-being. While often associated with mystics and monks, the essence of enlightenment has long been embedded across spiritual and philosophical traditions. It speaks to a universal longing: to understand oneself and one's place in the world, to live with clarity, and to experience inner peace.

Holistic health recognizes that true wellness includes not only the body but also the mind and spirit. When we explore enlightenment through this lens, it becomes less about dogma and more about the integration of awareness, connection, and personal transformation.

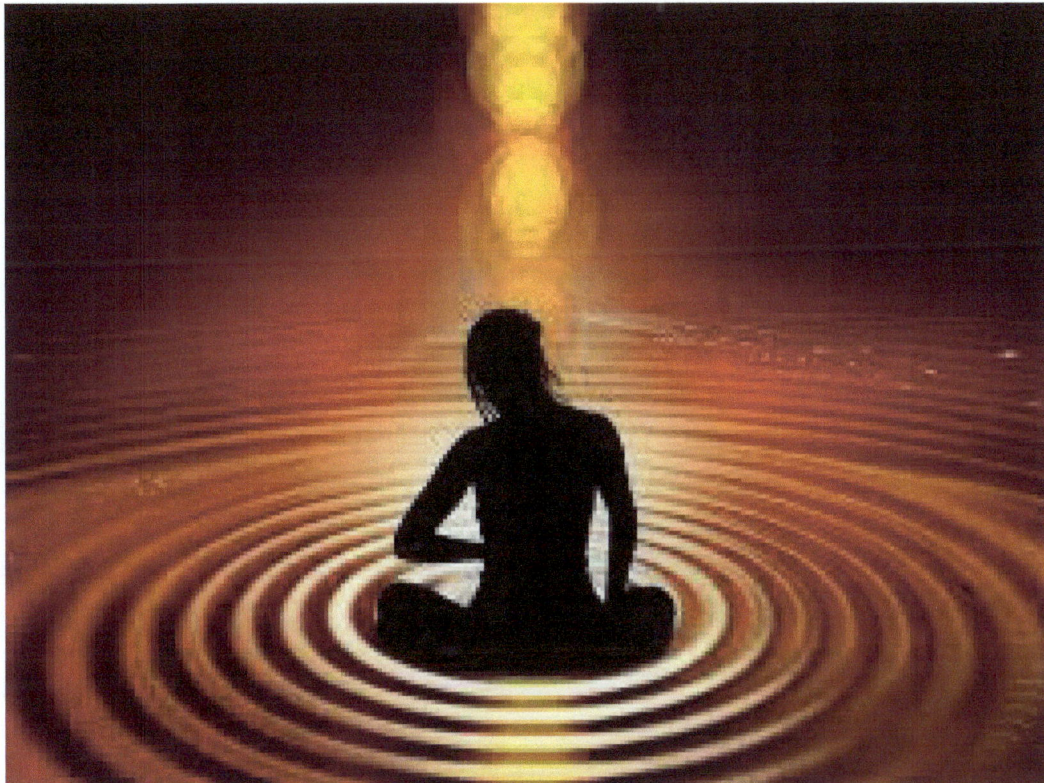

The Ancient Roots of Enlightenment: A Chronological Perspective
Across time and culture, humanity has reached for a transcendent state of wisdom and peace. Below is a historical look at how various traditions have been understood and named this experience:

1. Hinduism (c. 1500-1200 BCE)
Moksha refers to liberation from the cycle of rebirth (*samsara*) and the realization of one's oneness with the Absolute (*Brahman*). It emphasizes self-discipline, devotion, and philosophical inquiry-principles that resonate with today's holistic approaches to mindfulness and self-mastery.

2. Judaism (c. 1200-1000 BCE)

Devekut means "cleaving to God." It reflects an intense spiritual attachment and connection to the Divine, often nurtured through prayer, meditation on sacred texts, and acts of compassion. This mirrors modern interests in sacred ritual and spiritual intimacy within daily life.

3. Taoism (c. 600-400 BCE)

Wu Wei, or "effortless action," describes harmony with the *Tao*, or the natural order of the universe. It aligns beautifully with holistic living that promotes flow, simplicity, and balance through nature-based rhythms and minimalism.

4. Buddhism (c. 500 BCE)

Nirvana is the extinguishing of suffering, ignorance, and attachment. It is the ultimate liberation, discovered through the practice of mindfulness, ethical living, and meditative insight. *Bodhi*, or awakening, describes the experiential realization that leads to this state.

5. Christianity (c. 30 CE)

Illumination refers to the inner light that arises from divine communion. Practices like contemplative prayer, solitude, and service are paths to this inner radiance-echoing today's focus on stillness, presence, and soul care.

6. Islam (Sufism) (7th century CE)

Fana means the annihilation of the ego in the presence of God. In Sufi mysticism, it represents a deep surrender to divine love and truth-concepts that are increasingly embraced in emotional healing and ego work in holistic circles.

7. Sikhism (15th century CE)

Mukti signifies liberation from illusion and ego, and union with the Divine. It emphasizes selfless service, devotion, and equality principles foundational to both spiritual growth and community wellness.

8. New Age & Contemporary Spirituality (20th century CE onward)

Awakening / Self-Realization are the modern synthesis of East and West view of enlightenment as awakening to one's true nature. It often includes energy healing, intuitive development, and psychological integration-key aspects of the modern wellness movement.

b power thesaurus

Synonyms for Enlightenment

illumination   knowledge   education   insight

wisdom

Enlightenment and Holistic Wellness Today

In the context of holistic health, enlightenment is not about escaping the world. It's about engaging more deeply with it-intentionally, mindfully, and compassionately. Whether it's through yoga, mindful breathing, journaling, plant-based living, or spiritual inquiry, modern seekers are finding meaning in small, integrative practices that support mental clarity, emotional balance, and spiritual peace.

Importantly, enlightenment today is rarely seen as a final destination. Instead, it is a living process-a series of ongoing realizations and subtle shifts in consciousness. As individuals become more aware of their thoughts, behaviors, and purpose, they naturally align with states once reserved for sages and saints.

Why This Matters

In a time marked by information overload, stress, and disconnection, the timeless quest for enlightenment reminds us to return to our core. Holistic health is not just about the absence of disease-it is about the presence of meaning, clarity, compassion, and connection. Enlightenment, in all its cultural forms, is a call back to wholeness.

Whether you name it nirvana, moksha, awakening, or simply inner peace, the pursuit of higher awareness remains one of humanity's most enduring and necessary journeys.

A Holistic Look at Faith, Skepticism, and the Human Response to the Divine

Easter is one of the most widely celebrated religious holidays across the globe, observed by billions of people through both spiritual and cultural traditions. For Christians, it commemorates the resurrection of Jesus Christ, an event central to the faith and steeped in mystery, reverence, and awe. Yet, when we peel back the layers of devotion and ritual, deeper questions arise:

- What exactly happened leading up to the crucifixion?

- Why did Jesus die?

- If Jesus were alive today, would He be embraced or dismissed as a fraud?

- Would He be celebrated or condemned all over again?

These questions may seem theological at first glance, but they also probe into human psychology, sociology, and the nature of our collective consciousness. Let's explore this landscape more fully.

The Life and Death of Jesus: A Brief Chronology

The crucifixion of Jesus was not a random act of violence but the culmination of escalating tension. His teachings challenged the religious elite and threatened both Roman and Jewish political structures. Betrayed by Judas Iscariot, arrested in the Garden of Gethsemane, and denied three times by Peter, Jesus was ultimately condemned, scourged, and crucified under Roman law.

According to the Gospels, He died a slow, excruciating death, most likely from a combination of blood loss, asphyxiation, and shock. His body was placed in a tomb, and yet, three days later, reports of His resurrection spread. For the next 40 days, Jesus appeared to His disciples and followers in various places, teaching and preparing them before ascending into heaven.

But His post-resurrection appearances were not always public or easily verified, likely to avoid immediate conflict with His enemies. This subtle presence helped build the early Christian movement without triggering another wave of persecution, yet it also raises timeless questions.

Would Jesus Be Accepted Today?

Imagine Jesus walking the Earth today, preaching love, repentance, and divine truth. Would He be revered? Or ridiculed?

For many devout Christians, His return is not only expected but deeply hoped for. But it's also possible that His reappearance would challenge modern religious institutions, political ideologies, and cultural norms. His radical message of loving enemies, renouncing materialism, forgiving unconditionally, and living humbly runs counter to consumer culture, tribalism, and vengeance-based systems of justice.

In a secular and scientific age, He might be dismissed as delusional, cult-like, or mentally unstable. Social media would amplify both the adoration and the condemnation. News outlets would scrutinize every word. Authorities might intervene. Even some who claim to follow Him might not recognize Him if He failed to fit their expectations.

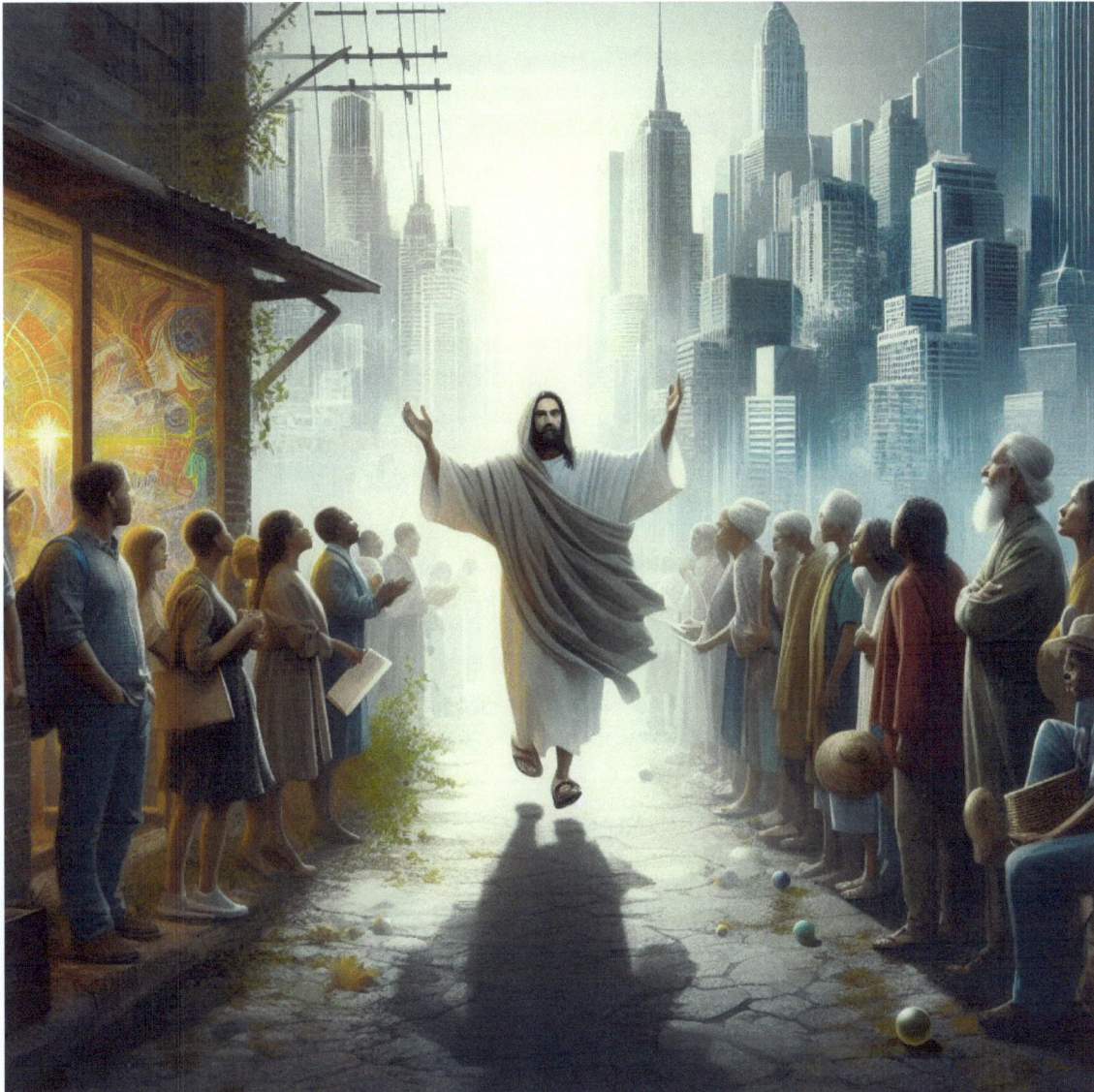

Miracles, Demons, and the Modern Lens

Jesus' time was filled with accounts of miracles such as healing the sick, calming storms, walking on water, and casting out demons. But how do we interpret those today?

It's worth asking: were demon possessions more common in antiquity, or was there simply a lack of medical and psychological understanding? Conditions we now label as epilepsy, schizophrenia, or PTSD may have once been seen through a spiritual lens. That doesn't necessarily disprove the spiritual dimension, it just reminds us that knowledge evolves, and perception is always shaped by context.

Many ancient cultures viewed health holistically, body, mind, and spirit as inseparable. In that light, Jesus' healing work can still be seen as deeply integrative, restoring not just physical health, but emotional, mental, and spiritual balance.

Do People Still Celebrate Easter as a Religious Holiday?

In the United States, Easter remains a significant holiday, but often more as a cultural celebration than a sacred observance. About 81% of Americans celebrate Easter (Statista, 2025), but only around 30% attend religious services (Jones, 2025). For many, Easter involves candy, egg hunts, spring fashion, and family meals more than deep spiritual reflection.

Globally, however, Easter remains a central pillar for over two billion Christians, and even those who don't consider themselves religious often participate in its communal and festive traditions.

The Pattern of Human Response to Visionaries

Jesus was not the only historical figure to be rejected in His time and revered later. In fact, history repeats itself with uncanny regularity (see chart ahead).

This pattern teaches us something vital: those who carry truth, challenge norms, or disrupt unjust systems are often rejected in their own time, only to be honored by future generations once the world has caught up.

Final Reflection

If Jesus Christ were to return today, not as a celebrity preacher or political figure, but as the humble, radical healer Jesus was, there's a strong chance he would face the same resistance that he did 2,000 years ago.

Yet, the holistic view reminds us that truth transcends time. While forms change, principles remain. Whether we view Jesus through a spiritual, symbolic, or historical lens, His life challenges us to look inward, to seek compassion, and to live from the soul rather than the ego.

The deeper question isn't whether the world would accept Jesus, but whether we would recognize Him in our own lives, our own thoughts, and the strangers we encounter daily.

References:

Statista. (2025, March 3). *Share of Americans celebrating Easter from 2009-2023*. https://www.statista.com/statistics/221108/share-of-americans-celebrating-easter-since-2007/

Jones, B. J. M. (2025, March 26). Church attendance has declined in most U.S. religious groups. Gallup.com. https://news.gallup.com/poll/642548/church-attendance-declined-religious-groups.aspx?utm_source=chatgpt.com

Figure	During Their Life	Now Remembered As
Jesus Christ	Executed as a criminal and heretic	Savior, Son of God, Redeemer
Socrates	Sentenced to death for corrupting the youth	Father of Western Philosophy
Martin Luther King Jr.	Monitored and opposed; assassinated	Civil Rights Icon
Joan of Arc	Burned at the stake for heresy	Catholic Saint and French Heroine
Galileo Galilei	Placed under house arrest for scientific beliefs	Father of Modern Science
Nelson Mandela	Imprisoned as a dissident	Global Symbol of Peace and Freedom
Mother Teresa	Criticized and praised	Canonized Saint and Humanitarian

Proverbs, *koans*, *dichos*, and *chengyu* are all concise expressions of cultural wisdom, yet they each emerge from unique linguistic and philosophical traditions. Though they may differ in form and function, they share the universal purpose of offering insight into human nature, behavior, and values. Below is a comparison that highlights their origins and distinctions.

Proverbs

- **Cultural Origin:** Found in virtually every language and culture worldwide, proverbs are traditional sayings passed down through generations.
- **Purpose:** Proverbs offer practical wisdom, moral lessons, or general truths about life. They are often metaphorical and easily remembered.
- **Examples:**
    - *"A stitch in time saves nine."*
    - *"Actions speak louder than words."*
    - *"Don't count your chickens before they hatch."*

Koans

- **Cultural Origin:** Originating in Chinese Chan Buddhism and further developed in Japanese Zen Buddhism, koans are used as a tool for spiritual training.
- **Purpose:** Koans are not meant to be logically solved. Instead, they challenge conventional reasoning and are used in meditation to provoke deep introspection and insight into the nature of self and reality.
- **Examples:**
    - *"What is the sound of one hand clapping?"*
    - *"What was your original face before your parents were born?"*

Dichos

- **Cultural Origin:** Common in the Spanish-speaking world, especially in Latin America and Spain, *dichos* are culturally rich sayings deeply embedded in Hispanic traditions.
- **Purpose:** Like proverbs, dichos reflect cultural values and offer observations or advice about life, often with regional flavor or humor.
- **Examples:**
    - *"No hay mal que por bien no venga"*
    (There's no bad from which good doesn't come.)
    - *"El que mucho abarca, poco aprieta"*
    (Jack of all trades, master of none.)

Chengyu

- **Cultural Origin:** Chengyu (成语) are idiomatic expressions from classical Chinese literature. Most consist of four characters and are rooted in historical or mythological events.
- **Purpose:** Chengyu condense complex narratives or moral lessons into brief, poetic form. They are often used in both written and spoken Chinese to convey layered meanings.
- **Examples:**
  - *卧薪尝胆* (wò xīn cháng dǎn) – *"To lie on firewood and taste gall."*
    Refers to enduring hardship and humiliation in pursuit of a goal or vengeance.
  - *画蛇添足* (huà shé tiān zú) – *"To draw legs on a snake."*
    Means to ruin something by overdoing it.

In summary, proverbs are universal sayings found in many cultures. Koans are paradoxical statements used in Zen Buddhism for meditation and self-realization. Dichos are Spanish-language proverbs commonly used in Hispanic cultures. Chenyus are from Chinese culture and are idiomatic expressions or set phrases. While they all share common goal of conveying wisdom, they vary in their cultural origins and specific uses.

From a holistic health perspective, such wisdom serves not only the intellect but the mind-body-spirit connection. These expressions often guide emotional balance, mindful behavior, and personal growth, cornerstones of overall well-being. They offer reminders of resilience, compassion, humility, and inner strength, supporting wellness not just as a state of physical health, but as a dynamic, cultural, and spiritual journey.

PROVERBS, KOANS, DICHOS and CHENGYU

PROVERBS	KOANS
Traditional sayings offering practical advice and general truths	Paradoxical statements for contemplation in Zen Buddhism
DICHOS	**CHENGYU**
Spanish-language expressions reflecting cultural values	Chinese idioms conveying complex ideas from lore

SECTION VI: Social Commentary & Group Psychology

My posts are mostly about holistic health, wellness, and various methods to achieve balance in our lives. Human behavior or psychology are subjects I have delved deeper into, as our behavior dramatically affects our mental, physical, and spiritual well-being.

The United States is a nation built on ideals of freedom, opportunity, and justice, but beneath these principles lies a web of contradictions. Many Americans know systemic issues, broken systems, and political dysfunction, yet they often feel powerless to enact meaningful change. Some believe they have no viable alternatives, while others simply don't care as long as the consequences don't affect them directly. Lack of agency (ability to act and make choices independently) and lack of control (exerting power or influence over others or outcomes) can have deep psychological effects, leading to many chronic cognitive ailments such as depression, anxiety, insecurity, and others. It's time for a collective reckoning. Perhaps it's time to ask not just, **"Are we part of the problem?"** but also, **"What can we do to be part of the solution?"**

COGNITIVE DISSONANCE

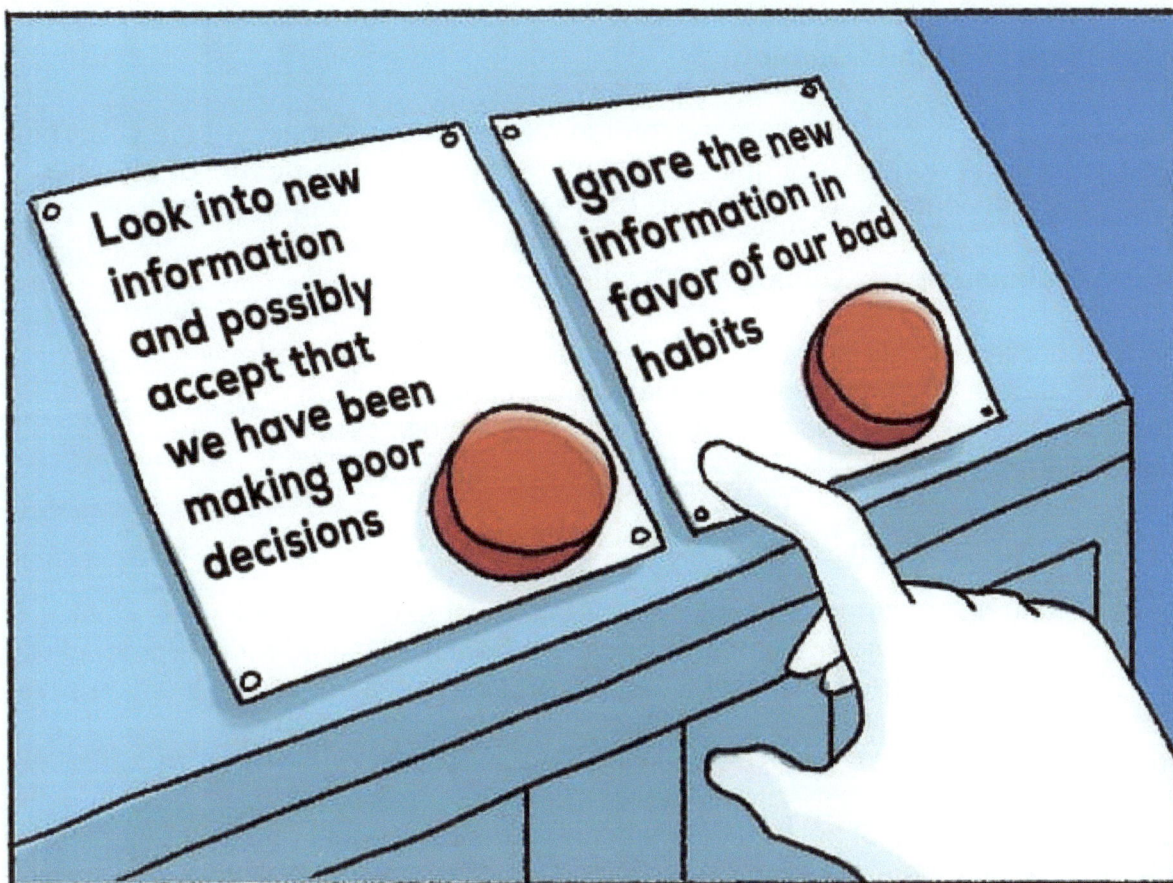

Here's a closer look at some of the most glaring contradictions or *cognitive dissonance* (the discomfort of holding conflicting beliefs or values) in American society, grouped by their interrelated themes:

🏛 Government and Political Dysfunction

1. Term Limits vs. Career Politicians

There is widespread support for imposing term limits on politicians, yet career politicians dominate Washington. Many Americans believe fresh perspectives would benefit governance, but efforts to enforce limits consistently stall. Voters complain about corruption but continue re-electing the same people.

2. Politicians and Insider Trading vs. Public Trust

Most Americans believe politicians should not benefit from insider trading, yet cases of elected officials profiting from privileged information persist. Despite this, the same politicians often get re-elected. We claim to detest corruption but keep endorsing those who abuse their positions.

3. Foreign Wars vs. Public Opinion

A large portion of the population opposes foreign military interventions, yet the U.S. remains entangled in conflicts worldwide. Public sentiment rarely translates into policy changes, highlighting the disconnect between the will of the people and government actions.

4. Perceived Misuse of Tax Dollars vs. Continued Compliance

Taxpayers express frustration over how their money is spent, with glaring examples of inefficiency and corruption. For instance, California spent $24 billion to address homelessness, yet the crisis has only worsened. Despite this, people continue paying taxes while feeling powerless to demand accountability.

5. Daylight Saving Time vs. Public Opinion

Twice a year, Americans grumble about the disruption caused by changing the clocks. Studies show that daylight saving time may increase health risks and reduce productivity, yet it persists. Despite widespread dissatisfaction, legislative inertia keeps the practice alive.

6. Limited Political Choices vs. Frustration with the Two-Party System

Americans lament the lack of political diversity and the stranglehold of the two-party system, yet alternative parties remain marginalized. Even though many feel disillusioned, they

146

continue to choose between the "lesser of two evils." Real change remains elusive because the system favors the status quo.

💰 Economics and Consumer Behavior

7. Support for Public Education vs. Private School Enrollment

Public education is hailed as the cornerstone of equal opportunity, yet families who can afford it often opt for private schooling. This creates a disconnect between advocating for public education and personal choices that contribute to inequality.

8. Supporting Local Businesses vs. Shopping Online

We talk about the importance of supporting local businesses, yet giants like Amazon, Walmart, and Starbucks continue to dominate, often putting small businesses out of business. Convenience, competitive pricing, and free shipping lure consumers away from their local economies.

9. Income Inequality vs. Celebrity Worship

While many decry income inequality and the wealth gap, America remains obsessed with celebrity culture and extravagant lifestyles. This fascination with the ultra-wealthy perpetuates distorted perceptions of success and value.

10. Perceived Value vs. Price Sensitivity

Consumers often complain about the declining quality of goods and services but continue purchasing cheap, mass-produced items instead of supporting higher-quality alternatives. The desire for instant gratification and low prices outweighs long-term sustainability.

🏥 Health, Lifestyle, and Well-Being

11. Fast Food Consumption vs. Health Awareness

We know fast food is unhealthy. Obesity rates continue to soar, yet fast-food chains thrive. Parents claim they care about their children's health but often default to convenience, feeding them processed foods while allowing endless hours of screen time. Nutrition takes a backseat to ease, and the consequences are generational.

12. Sedentary Lifestyles vs. Advocacy for Healthy Living

We advocate for fitness, movement, and healthy living, yet modern lifestyles promote sedentary habits—long hours at desks, excessive screen time, and minimal physical activity. Knowledge doesn't always translate to action.

13. Healthcare System Criticism vs. Reliance on It

Americans recognize that the healthcare system is broken, yet they remain reliant on it. Pharmaceutical companies flood media with advertisements, influencing consumers and doctors alike. The system favors profits over people, but viable alternatives are scarce, leaving many trapped in a cycle of dependency.

14. Body Positivity vs. Unrealistic Beauty Standards

The body positivity movement advocates for acceptance and inclusivity, but media, advertising, and Hollywood continue to promote unrealistic beauty standards. Thinness, youth, and perfection remain the ideal, perpetuating negative body image and self-esteem issues.

15. Desire for Work-Life Balance vs. Overworking Culture

Many Americans yearn for a better work-life balance, yet the culture of overwork persists. Long hours, limited vacation time, and a "hustle mentality" lead to burnout and mental health struggles. We value personal well-being in theory but often sacrifice it in practice.

🌍 Environment and Sustainability

16. Environmental Awareness vs. Consumerism

Many Americans express concern about climate change and environmental degradation but continue consuming at unsustainable levels. Convenience, affordability, and habit often override sustainable choices. The "Not in My Backyard" (NIMBY) mentality prevails, as people want solutions without altering their lifestyles.

17. Recycling Rhetoric vs. Minimal Action

Americans advocate for recycling and environmental protection, yet most recycling programs are underutilized or ineffective. Many items placed in recycling bins end up in landfills, and people often lack awareness of proper recycling practices.

🔒 Privacy, Technology, and Social Isolation

18. Privacy Concerns vs. Social Media Addiction

Many express concerns over privacy and data security in the digital age, yet millions willingly share intimate details of their lives on platforms that harvest personal data. We fear surveillance but continue scrolling, liking, and posting. Convenience and entertainment often outweigh the fear of losing control over our private information.

19. Spam, Telemarketers, and Privacy Violations vs. Acceptance of Invasions

Americans complain about the relentless onslaught of spam calls, telemarketers, and digital intrusions, yet many accept these invasions as a normal part of modern life. We express frustration over privacy violations but rarely take steps to secure our information or demand accountability from corporations that exploit personal data.

20. Community Engagement vs. Social Isolation
Americans value community engagement and connection, yet the rise of digital communication and urbanization has led to increased social isolation. We crave connection but often retreat into virtual worlds, losing the sense of belonging that real communities provide. We see electronic devices as babysitters for children and adults alike, and then wonder why so many are depressed, anxious, and unable to be comfortable in real-life social settings.

21. Mistrust of Big Tech vs. Dependence on It

Americans frequently express mistrust of big tech companies, citing concerns about monopolies, privacy, and censorship. Yet, dependence on platforms like Google, Facebook, and Amazon remains pervasive. We resent their power but rely on their convenience.

⚖️ Ethics, Morality, and Social Justice

22. Human Rights Advocacy vs. Selective Outrage

Many advocate for human rights and justice but remain selective in their outrage, often influenced by political affiliations or cultural biases. Genuine concern for equality should transcend partisanship, yet inconsistencies persist.

23. Religious Values vs. Material Pursuits

America prides itself on being a nation of faith, yet materialism and consumerism often overshadow spiritual values. Many profess religious beliefs but prioritize wealth, status, and success over moral and ethical principles.

24. Public Demand for Change vs. Fear of Disruption

Perhaps the most significant contradiction is that while Americans express a desire for change, they also fear the disruption that change may bring. Breaking free from familiar systems requires effort, sacrifice, and discomfort—something many are unwilling to endure.

25. The Forgotten Victims: Native Americans and Historical Amnesia

America celebrates its history of freedom and democracy while ignoring the ongoing consequences of genocide and displacement inflicted on Native American communities. Treaties were broken, lands were stolen, and entire cultures were nearly erased. Yet, mainstream narratives often gloss over these atrocities, perpetuating historical amnesia. The plight of Native Americans remains a footnote in history books, even as they continue to face systemic inequalities.

26. Advocacy for Social Justice vs. Ignoring Indigenous Struggles

While advocating for social justice and equality, many overlook the ongoing struggles of indigenous communities. Issues such as land sovereignty, environmental degradation, and broken treaties remain unresolved, highlighting a glaring inconsistency in America's commitment to justice.

🔍 A Nation at a Crossroads

America's contradictions are not just individual dilemmas—they reflect the collective psyche of a nation grappling with competing values and desires. To move forward, we must confront these inconsistencies with honesty and courage. True change starts not just by acknowledging these contradictions but by taking deliberate action to align our values with our behavior. *"Change the world!" "Fix the system!"*

Instead: Are we ready to face the mirror? How about changing ourselves?

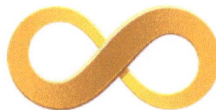

∞

The Role and Risks of Closed Social Groups in Martial Arts, Yoga, Clubs, and Other Exclusive Communities

Closed social groups, such as private yoga or martial arts schools, serve a unique purpose within their respective disciplines. Depending on the intent behind their structure, their exclusivity can have advantages and drawbacks. Similar dynamics can be found in other exclusive communities, such as religious orders, secret societies, and elite academic circles.

Advantages of Closed Groups

1. **Focused Learning Environment**
   - By restricting access, students or members can focus on their objectives without outside distractions or feeling self-conscious under public scrutiny. This is particularly important for traditional martial arts, esoteric yoga practices, or spiritual communities that require deep practices of observation, contemplation, and meditation as their main focus.
2. **Preservation of Tradition**
   - Many closed schools and societies follow lineages that prioritize secrecy or direct transmission from teacher to student. This can help to maintain authenticity, ensuring knowledge isn't diluted or misrepresented.
3. **Community and Trust**
   - A closed structured system can encourage a strong sense of belonging, loyalty, and trust among members. This is very important for practices that involve partner training, deep introspection, or energy work, as well as in religious and esoteric orders.
4. **Safety and Progression**
   - Some disciplines involve physical conditioning or internal energy cultivation such as with advanced qigong, martial techniques, or breath control methods. Restricting access ensures students have proper guidance and do not attempt techniques without foundational preparation.

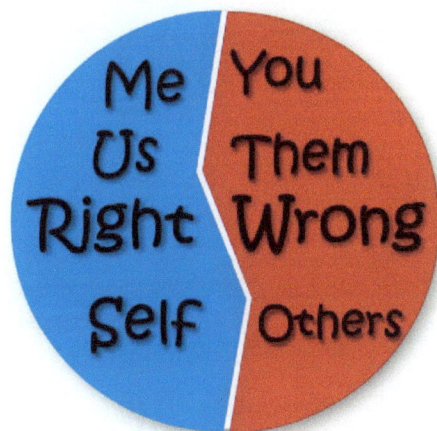

CLOSED SOCIAL GROUPS

Healthy "Open Structure"
Strictly "Closed Structure"

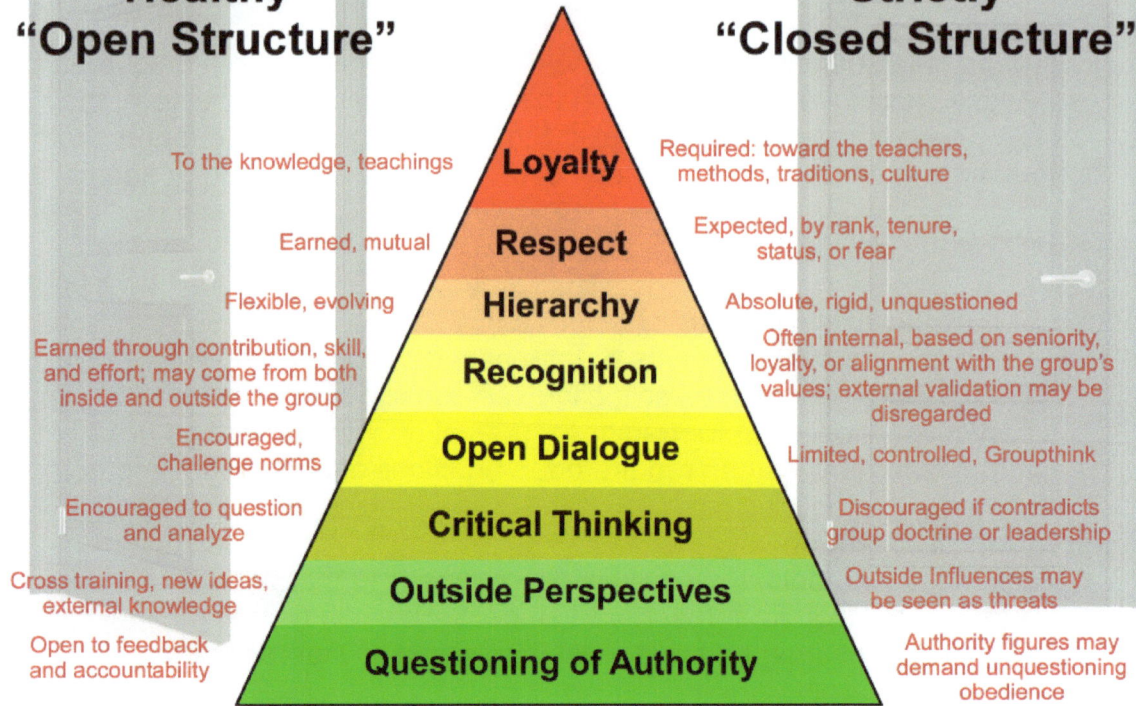

	Healthy "Open Structure"	Strictly "Closed Structure"
Loyalty	To the knowledge, teachings	Required: toward the teachers, methods, traditions, culture
Respect	Earned, mutual	Expected, by rank, tenure, status, or fear
Hierarchy	Flexible, evolving	Absolute, rigid, unquestioned
Recognition	Earned through contribution, skill, and effort; may come from both inside and outside the group	Often internal, based on seniority, loyalty, or alignment with the group's values; external validation may be disregarded
Open Dialogue	Encouraged, challenge norms	Limited, controlled, Groupthink
Critical Thinking	Encouraged to question and analyze	Discouraged if contradicts group doctrine or leadership
Outside Perspectives	Cross training, new ideas, external knowledge	Outside Influences may be seen as threats
Questioning of Authority	Open to feedback and accountability	Authority figures may demand unquestioning obedience

www.MindandBodyExercises.com

© Copyright 2025 CAD Graphics, Inc.

Potential Disadvantages

1. **Exclusivity Can Limit Growth**
   - While privacy may support depth, it may also prevent potential new students from finding and benefiting from these practices. A highly restricted group may unintentionally create an echo chamber.

2. **Loss of Cultural Exchange**
   - Martial arts, yoga, and many esoteric traditions have deep historical roots but have evolved through cultural exchange. Over-restricting access could hinder the natural development of these traditions.

3. **Risk of Elitism or Dogmatism**
   - If not managed well, closed groups can sometimes lead to rigid, authoritarian-type hierarchies, where senior members become resistant to new ideas or outsiders. This can lead to stagnation rather than growth.

4. **Barrier to Understanding**
   - In some cases, secrecy can lead to stigma, misinformation, or misinterpretation from outsiders of the group who speculate about what happens within the group.

When Closed Groups Use Insular Dynamics

Closed groups, whether in martial arts, yoga, religious sects, secret societies, or elite academic circles, can sometimes encourage an "us vs. them" mentality, especially if they become overly insular. Various terms refer to these types of groups such as, but not limited to:

- **Dogmatic Communities**
- **Ideological Isolation**
- **Rigid Group Mentality**
- **Sectarian Influence**
- **Closed-System Thinking**
- **Insulated Hierarchies**
- **Excessive Group Loyalty**
- **Echo Chamber Environments**
- **Insular Traditions**
- **Cult-like**

Groupthink & Echo Chambers

- Critical or objective thinking can diminish in highly insular groups as members conform to a singular worldview.
- If a martial arts school, spiritual order, or elite academic group never question its methods, or principles or refuses outside perspectives, it risks stagnation, stigma, and dogma.
- Some groups discourage members from engaging with alternative viewpoints, reinforcing a "this is the only way" mindset.

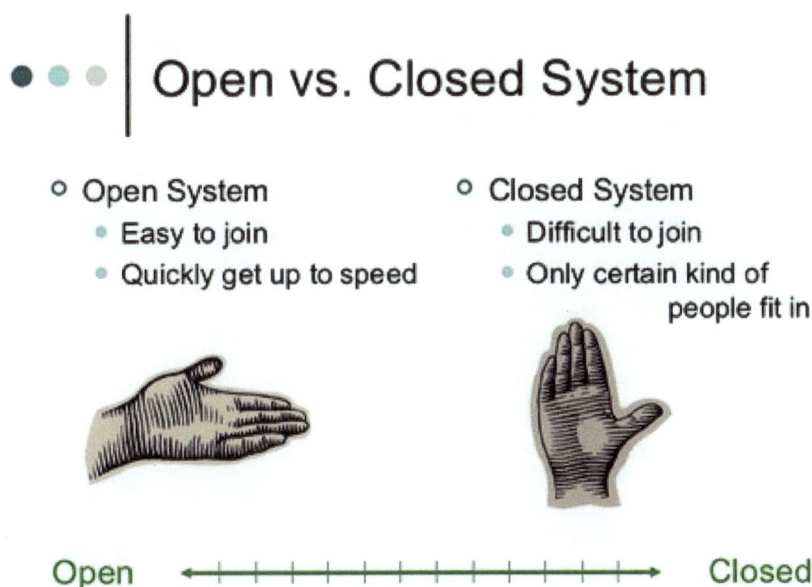

● ● ● | Open vs. Closed System

○ Open System
  • Easy to join
  • Quickly get up to speed

○ Closed System
  • Difficult to join
  • Only certain kind of people fit in

Open ←——————————————→ Closed

Isolationism & "Us vs. Them" Mentality

- If those outside of the group are viewed with hesitation, suspicion, or unworthiness, the group can become exclusionary rather than welcoming.
- Some esoteric circles, religious sects, or martial arts schools forbid interactions with non-members, creating psychological dependence.
- Over time, this can erode personal autonomy and discourage critical reflection.

Loaded Language & Indoctrination

- Exclusive terminology or redefined words, such as "true knowledge," "higher-level students," "the only," the original," etc., can create a psychological barrier between insiders and outsiders.
- Language may be used to elevate the in-group while dismissing external knowledge as inferior, dangerous or subversive.
- In more extreme cases, dissenting members may be labeled as "unenlightened," "not loyal," "not ready," "not qualified," or "not clear" to justify exclusion.

Leader Worship & Hierarchical Control

- Some martial arts or yoga masters, religious leaders, or academic figures present themselves as the sole gatekeeper of knowledge, discouraging students or disciples from questioning authority.
- Strict obedience without space for personal growth can create an authoritarian dynamic, where members fear questioning the instructor, leader or those in authority.
- This is especially risky in some of the internal arts and esoteric traditions, where progress is subjective and can be manipulated through metaphysical, mystical or vague claims.

How to Avoid or Become Aware of Insular Dynamics in Closed Groups

- **Encourage Critical Thinking:** Healthy groups welcome questions and debate rather than discouraging independent thought.
- **Allow Cross-Training and Exchange:** Exposure to other traditions, teachers, perspectives and resources keeps members from falling into dogma.
- **Maintain Ethical Boundaries:** If the group expects extreme devotion, secrecy, or control over members' lives, it's a huge red flag.
- **Avoid Fear-Based Loyalty:** No legitimate school or organization should use fear, guilt, or manipulation to keep members from leaving.
- **Foster Openness Without Dilution:** A "semi-closed model," where serious training is protected but knowledge is not hoarded, may be able to better balance tradition with accessibility.

US versus THEM

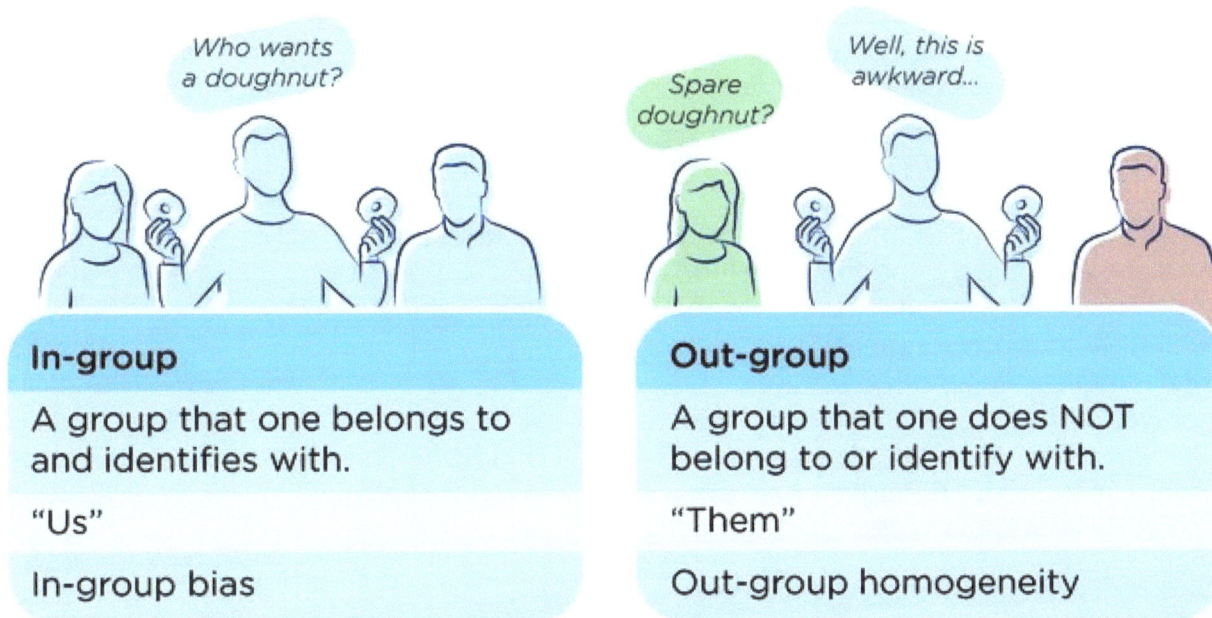

In-group
A group that one belongs to and identifies with.

"Us"

In-group bias

Out-group
A group that one does NOT belong to or identify with.

"Them"

Out-group homogeneity

Jack Westin

Are Closed Groups Always Bad?

Not necessarily. Some amount of exclusivity can be beneficial for:

☑ Protecting advanced knowledge from misuse
☑ Maintaining depth and focus while training
☑ Creating a dedicated, distraction-free environment

However, if a group starts demanding absolute loyalty, rejecting all outsiders, or discouraging independent thinking, then it risks cult-like tendencies. Striking a balance between exclusivity and openness is key to ensuring that these groups remain places of learning, growth, and genuine tradition rather than echo chambers of control and manipulation.

With over 20 years of firsthand experience training, studying, and teaching in various closed groups across different settings, I have observed both their strengths and challenges. I then dedicated an additional 25 years to studying the underlying dynamics that shape these environments, recognizing both their positive and negative consequences. To deepen my understanding, I further invested four years into the study of psychology, religion, Eastern philosophy, sociology, psychophysiology, and other related fields, allowing me to analyze closed group behavior with a broader and more informed perspective.

Why Even Highly Educated Professionals Fall for Misinformation

As someone who has spent over four decades practicing, studying, and teaching martial arts and holistic health, I have witnessed firsthand the gradual erosion of authenticity and deception in traditional practices, particularly in the United States. With a Bachelor of Science in Holistic Health and formal studies in psychology, sociology, PTSD, physiopsychology, religion, philosophy, Eastern thought, and the U.S. healthcare system, I have sought to understand why deception in professional and educational settings is so prevalent. Beyond martial arts, my experience includes 20 years at a high level within a highly insular, strongly hierarchical, and ideologically rigid organization that fostered a deeply immersive and echo-chamber environment. Within this structure, dogmatic teachings were reinforced, and critical inquiry was often discouraged. These insights have given me firsthand exposure to the power of groupthink, social conditioning, and blind trust in authority, leading me to question why even highly educated professionals, those who pride themselves on knowledge and integrity can fall for deceptive practices, sometimes unknowingly, sometimes willingly.

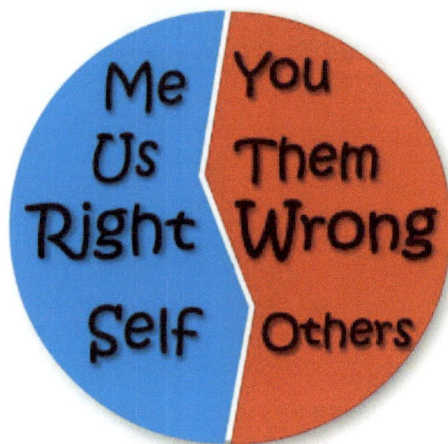

The answer lies in a mix of psychological phenomena, social conditioning, and systemic complacency, all of which contribute to the uncritical acceptance of misinformation and misrepresented traditions.

How Deception Manifests in Professional Circles

The Bait-and-Switch Model

A classic example of deception is called the "bait-and-switch" model, or the practice of marketing one thing while delivering something entirely different.

In martial arts, particularly tai chi, many instructors advertise lineage-based training but actually teach a mix of simplified qigong movements that lack the biomechanical structure,

156

martial application, and philosophical depth of true tai chi. This bait-and-switch is not always done with malice, sometimes, these instructors were themselves misled.

The same pattern occurs in healthcare, education, and professional training programs. A wellness coach may be certified in "tai chi" after a weekend workshop that teaches nothing more than generic breathing exercises. A doctor might recommend a therapeutic method without investigating its legitimacy, relying solely on institutional backing.

Why does this happen? Because highly educated individuals are just as susceptible to deception as anyone else, sometimes even more so.

Understanding how misinformation spreads among professionals requires a closer examination of the psychological mechanisms at play. Many assume that education alone is enough to safeguard against deception, but the reality is more complex. The intersection of cognitive biases, institutional structures, and social pressures creates an environment where even well-meaning professionals may unknowingly perpetuate falsehoods.

COMMON EXAMPLES OF **COGNITIVE BIAS**

Assuming that our own judgments and beliefs are always correct

Attributing other people's success to luck or external factors

Failing to actively seek out objective facts and instead relying on limited or biased information

Trusting someone more based on their perceived authority or status

Constantly blaming others when things don't go their way

Assuming that everyone shares the same opinion and belief

Using mental shortcuts or simplified strategies in decision-making

MIND HELP

MINDJOURNAL

Psychological Mechanisms That Enable Deception

1. Groupthink and Echo Chambers

Groupthink occurs when individuals prioritize group cohesion over critical thinking. In professional circles, questioning widely accepted practices can be socially and professionally risky. If an institution, hospital, or wellness center endorses a particular method, many professionals will blindly accept it rather than challenge its legitimacy.

Similarly, echo chambers are where people are only exposed to information that reinforces their beliefs, creating an illusion of consensus. In other words, if "everyone" in the field is saying something is true, then it must be, right?

Example: A hospital integrates "tai chi" into patient care, but what they are actually promoting is a set of disconnected qigong exercises. Because multiple institutions endorse the same program, no one questions its authenticity.

2. Compliance and Institutional Authority

Many professionals trust authority figures and institutions over personal investigation. If a method is backed by a well-known organization, it is often assumed to be legitimate. Compliance within hierarchical structures, such as hospitals, universities, or corporate training programs, discourages critical inquiry.

Another crucial factor is the *Dunning-Kruger Effect*, where individuals with limited knowledge overestimate their competence. This is particularly problematic in fields where professionals receive superficial training in a subject yet assume they have mastered it. A healthcare provider who attends a weekend seminar on tai chi, for example, may believe they fully grasp its principles and applications, despite lacking the years of rigorous training required for true expertise. This misplaced confidence can lead them to misrepresent tai chi, endorse incorrect practices, or dismiss criticisms from those with deeper knowledge.

Example: A university offers a "Tai Chi for Rehabilitation" certification, but the course is taught by individuals with no connection to lineage-based tai chi. Students accept the curriculum as valid because it comes from an academic institution.

The Dunning-Kruger Effect

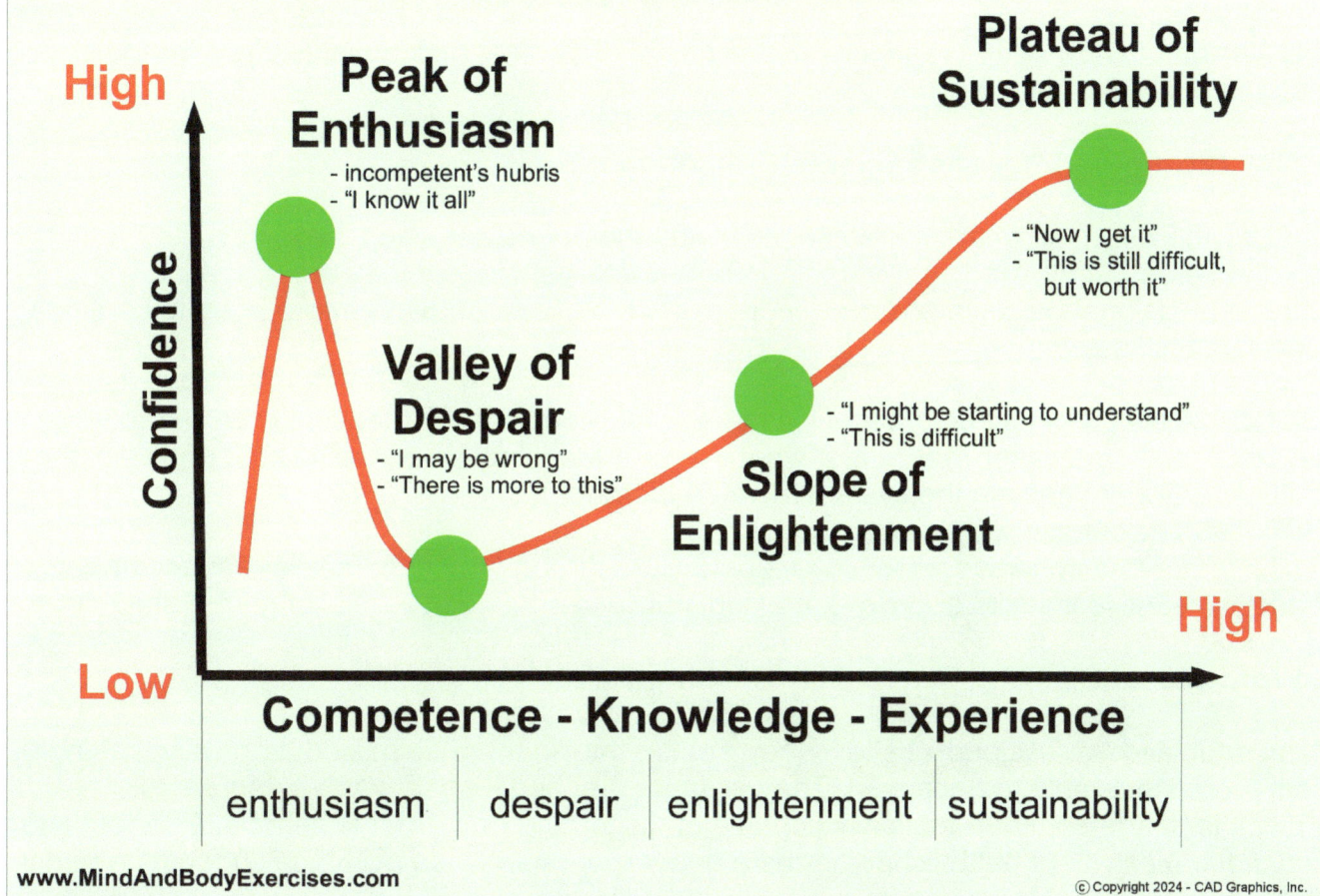

High

Confidence

Peak of Enthusiasm
- incompetent's hubris
- "I know it all"

Plateau of Sustainability
- "Now I get it"
- "This is still difficult, but worth it"

Valley of Despair
- "I may be wrong"
- "There is more to this"

Slope of Enlightenment
- "I might be starting to understand"
- "This is difficult"

High

Low

Competence - Knowledge - Experience

| enthusiasm | despair | enlightenment | sustainability |

www.MindAndBodyExercises.com © Copyright 2024 - CAD Graphics, Inc.

3. Cognitive Dissonance and The Need to Justify Investment

Cognitive dissonance occurs when individuals experience psychological discomfort due to conflicting beliefs. Rather than admit they were misled, they will often rationalize their choices.

Example: A doctor who has been teaching "tai chi" to patients later discovers that what they learned has no real connection to tai chi principles. Instead of acknowledging the error, they convince themselves that what they teach is "good enough" because patients seem to benefit from it.

The greater the investment, whether in time, money, or personal reputation, the harder it becomes to admit fault.

4. Loss of Agency and The Illusion of Knowledge
Loss of agency happens when people rely too much on external validation rather than personal research. Many professionals believe that because they are educated, they are immune to deception, a form of bias of overconfidence.

159

Example: A physical therapist learns tai chi from a single continuing education course and assumes they now "know" tai chi. They never think to seek a lineage-based teacher because they believe their credentials alone make them competent.

This illusion of knowledge creates a false sense of expertise, making individuals less likely to seek out authentic sources.

5. The Hawthorne Effect and Operant Conditioning

The *Hawthorne Effect* refers to people modifying their behavior when they know they are being observed, often leading them to reinforce whatever system they are operating within. When professionals receive positive feedback for their work, they are more likely to continue it, even if it is flawed.

Example: A wellness instructor receives praise and recognition for teaching "tai chi" to seniors. Even if they later realize that what they are teaching lacks real tai chi principles, they continue anyway because the system rewards them for it.

Similarly, *operant conditioning* reinforces behaviors through rewards (career advancement, financial incentives, social approval), making individuals hesitant to challenge the status quo.

6. Professional Bias and Status Quo Thinking

Many educated professionals believe they are too intelligent to be misled, ironically making them more vulnerable to deception. They assume that because they have degrees or certifications, they are automatically capable of discerning truth from falsehood. This leads to *status quo bias* where established norms are favored, even when evidence suggests a better alternative.

Example: A medical board endorses a "tai chi" program without verifying its authenticity. Because it is institutionally approved, healthcare professionals continue promoting it even if they suspect it is inaccurate.

The Responsibility of Professionals to Seek Truth

Highly educated individuals, especially those who interact with the public, must be held to a higher standard of due diligence. Their decisions impact patients, students, and clients, and therefore, they have an ethical obligation to verify the accuracy of what they promote. While many professionals fall for misinformation unintentionally, willful ignorance is not an excuse. In an era where information is readily available, professionals should be expected to:

- Question the validity of institutional endorsements.

- Seek primary sources and traditional lineages when applicable.

- Acknowledge and correct misinformation rather than doubling down on errors.

Failure to do so not only undermine their credibility but also erodes public trust in education, healthcare, and martial arts traditions.

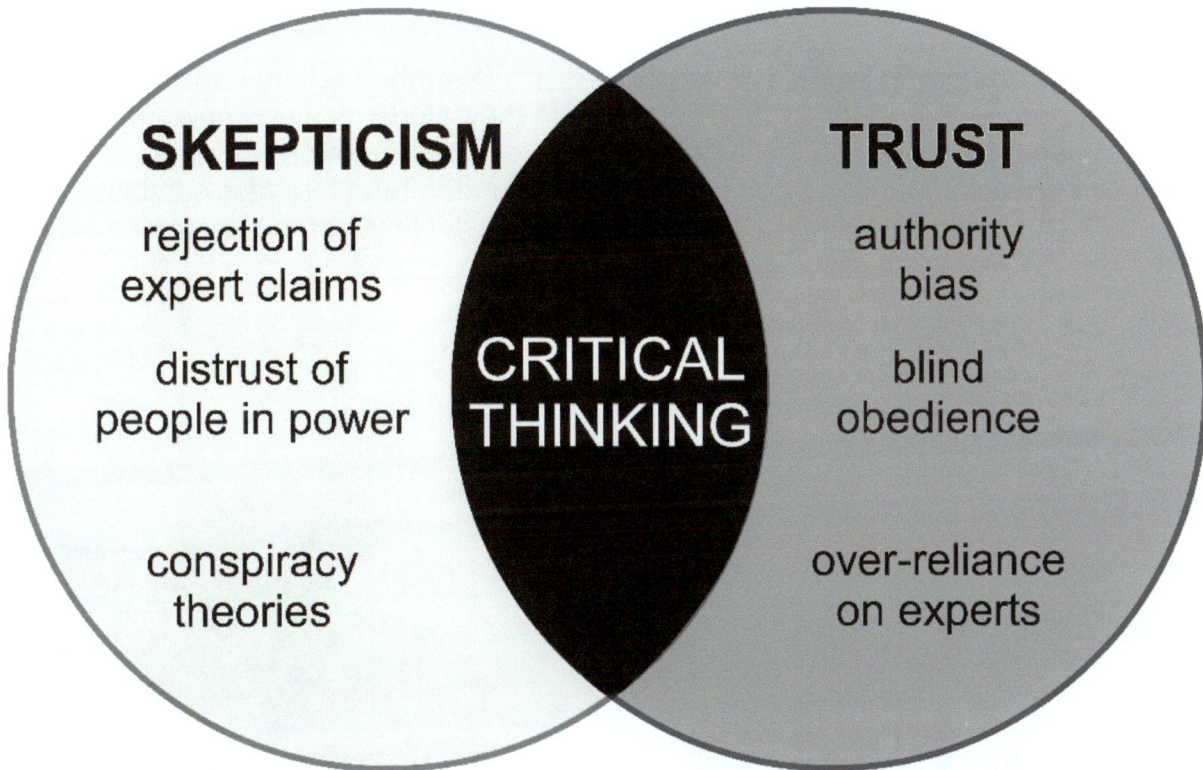

Conclusion: A Call for Intellectual Integrity

Deception in martial arts, healthcare, and other fields is not just an individual issue. It is a systemic problem rooted in cognitive biases, institutional authority, and social conditioning. By understanding the psychological mechanisms behind why professionals fall for misinformation, we can begin to challenge these patterns and restore integrity to our disciplines.

Education should not be about blind acceptance, but rather it should be about critical inquiry, truth-seeking, and personal responsibility. Those who pride themselves on knowledge must be willing to go beyond surface-level expertise and seek the depth that true mastery requires.

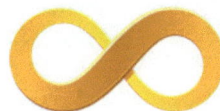

Opening the Circle: How Wise Educators Welcome Outside Insight

As someone who has spent a lifetime immersed in holistic health, martial arts, qigong, and Eastern traditions, and authored 30 books on these subjects, I've encountered a curious dynamic when trying to share my work with fellow educators, programs, and organizations in the field.

Some colleagues and group leaders have wholeheartedly embraced my books, integrating them into their programs and recommending them to their students as complementary resources. These individuals and institutions see value in offering a broader lens and deeper tools, without fear of comparison or competition. They understand that true education isn't about controlling a student's learning but about nurturing it. However, not everyone responds this way.

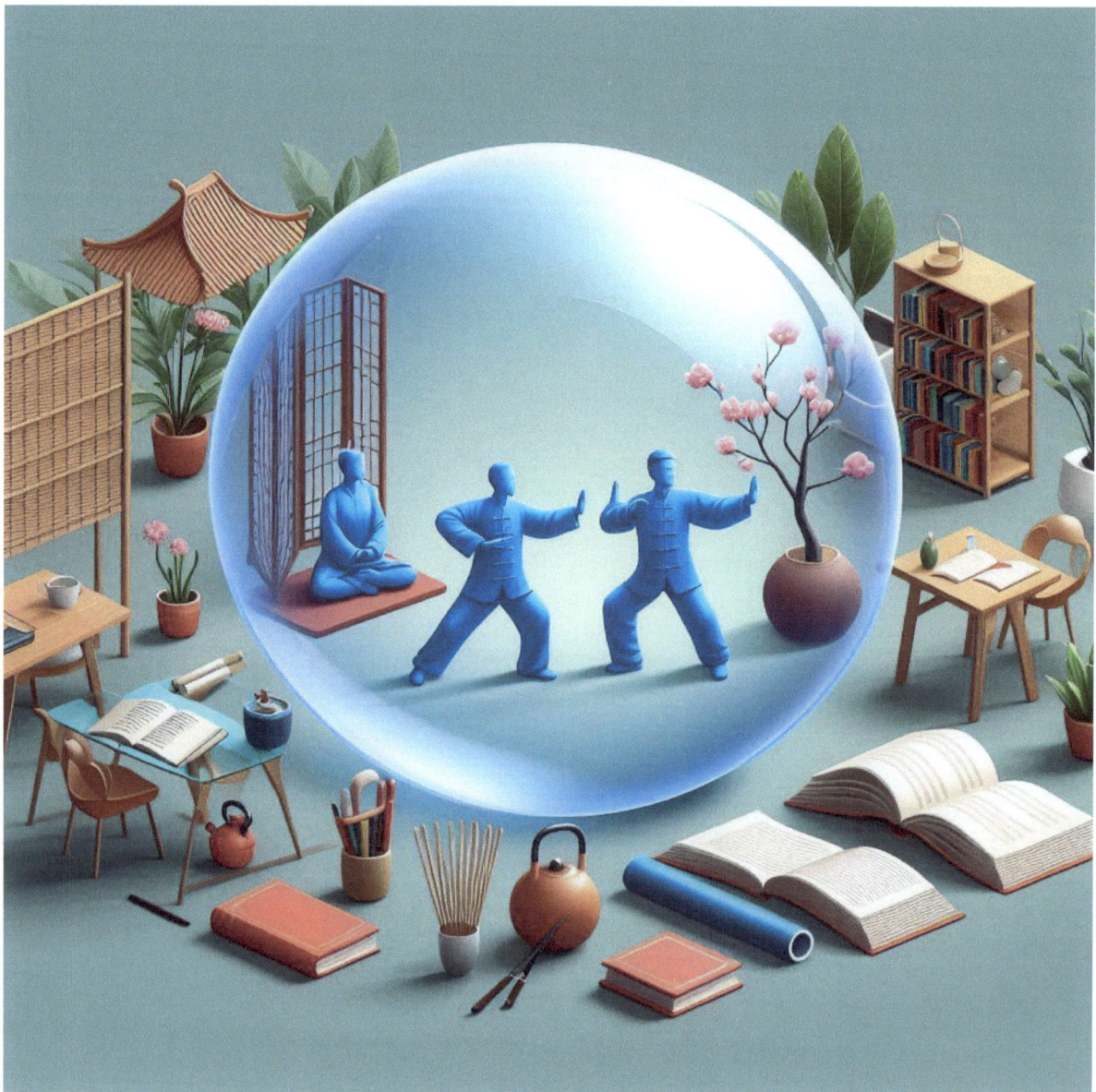

Some instructors, schools, and even entire systems appear hesitant to recommend or promote my work and that of others outside of their bubble. In certain cases, there seems to be an unspoken fear. A fear that perhaps their students will see gaps in their own curriculum or discover new or more complete skills and insights not offered in their current learning path. It's as though by acknowledging an external source of knowledge, they feel their authority or cohesion might be challenged.

This has raised an important question, that others working in fields of mastery and personal development may also face:

How do we navigate the tension between sharing our work and respecting the insecurities it may awaken in others?

Ego in the Path of Learning

In the very traditions many of us teach, ego is framed as the primary obstacle to growth. Yet even in practices designed to transcend ego, such as tai chi, meditation, and internal martial arts, ego often remains hidden in plain sight. A teacher or institution may subtly discourage external learning, not because the material lacks value, but because they feel exposed or threatened by it.

The deeper truth is this: a student's growth should never be seen as a threat to a teacher's role or a program's identity. If anything, it's a testament to the strength of their foundational guidance. When leaders cling to authority at the expense of their students' evolution, they ultimately hinder the very progress their mission was meant to support.

The Role of Loyalty and Closed Systems

Another dimension that often goes unspoken is the role of *loyalty.* A quality that, while admirable, can sometimes limit a student's growth when tied to overly hierarchical or ideologically rigid systems.

In some organizations, students are immersed in highly structured environments where authority is concentrated, hierarchies are strict, and questioning the curriculum is discouraged. These groups often cultivate a deep sense of allegiance, whether to a teacher, lineage, ideology, or system. This loyalty can create a powerful psychological barrier, making students feel that seeking information elsewhere is a form of betrayal.

When this dynamic becomes dominant, students may become hesitant to explore new resources, even when those resources are directly aligned with their path of growth. Out of respect or fear, they remain in a tightly controlled learning environment, sometimes unaware of how limited their exposure has become.

This kind of immersion often leads to echo chambers, where the same concepts, styles, and interpretations are reinforced over and over. While repetition is a valid and often necessary method of training, when it replaces diversity of thought and cross-pollination of ideas, the result is stagnation, both intellectually and spiritually.

From Competition to Collaboration

The mindset that views another's work as a threat is rooted in scarcity: the idea that there's only so much wisdom, attention, or recognition to go around. But those of us who have walked these paths know better. Real mastery breeds humility and a sense of abundance. There is always more to explore, more to share, and more to co-create together.

That's why I've shifted my focus toward collaboration with those who operate from an open, growth-oriented paradigm. To teachers, schools, organizations, and systems that view education as a dynamic and shared mission, and not a personal or ideological pedestal. These "out of the box" thinkers are actively transforming how knowledge is shared, empowering their students with rich, multidimensional resources that enhance the learning journey.

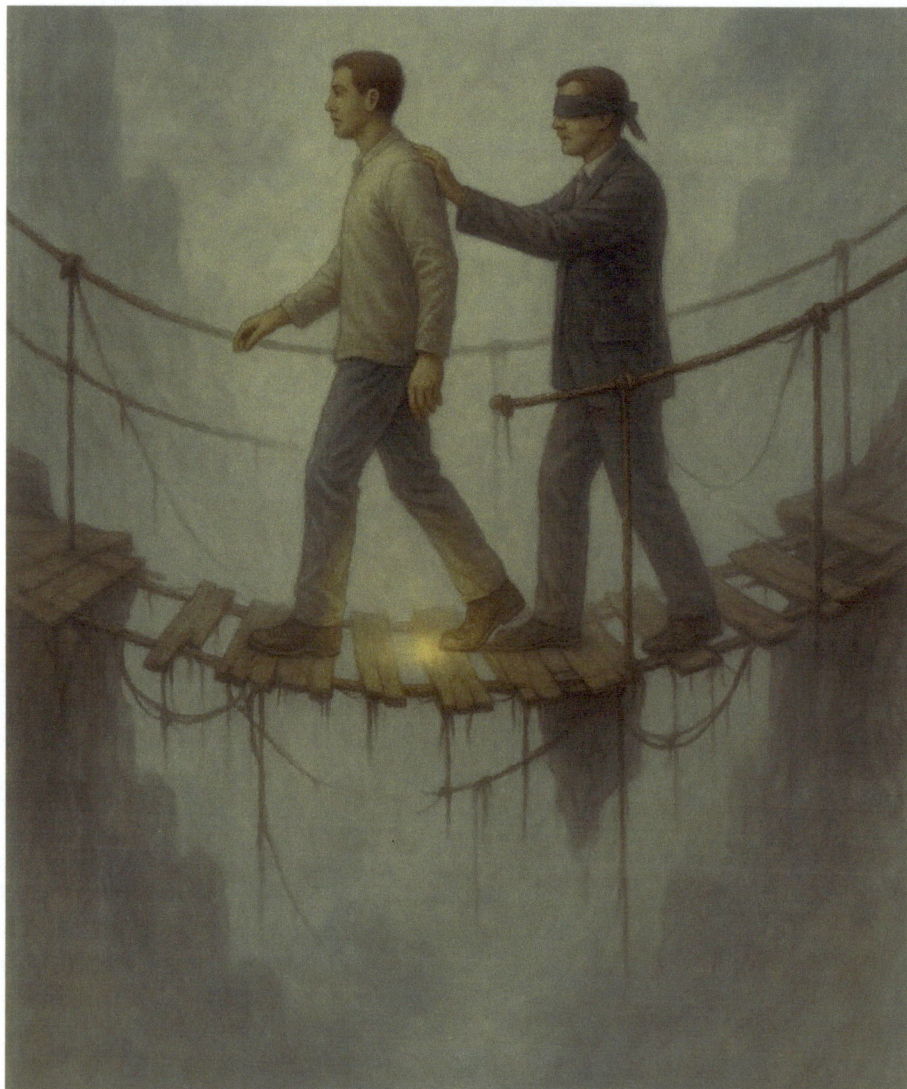

Reframing the Message

To support this shift, I've worked to frame my books as teaching companions, not replacements. They're meant to enhance the student experience, deepen understanding of nuanced principles, and provide historical and philosophical context that may not fit into the rhythm of regular classes or structured programs.

Some schools and instructors have even offered to write forewords for custom editions or bundle my books into their recommended reading lists, helping students understand how the material supports, not replaces their core instruction.

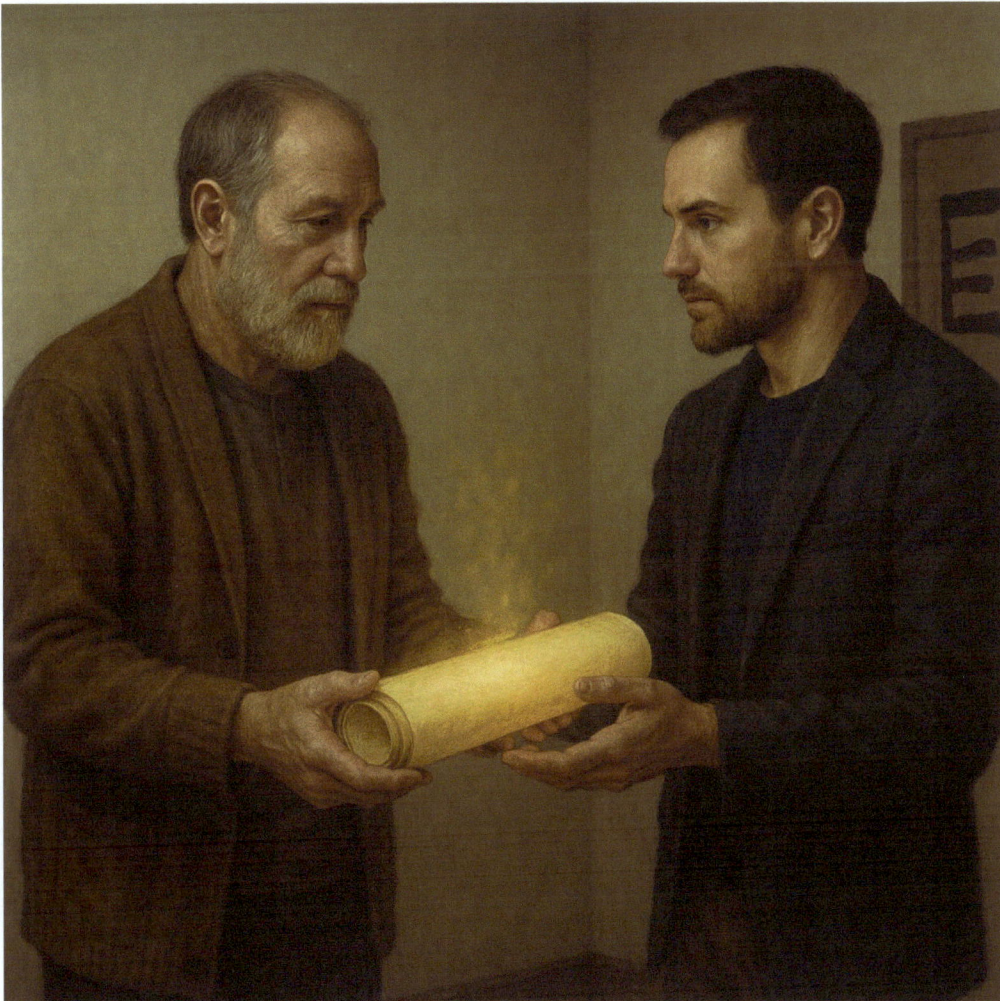

Creating Supportive Alliances

Rather than positioning my work as something to be adopted with hesitation, I aim to foster supportive alliances or mutual relationships with like-minded educators and organizations who are excited about sharing resources for the benefit of the student body. This spirit of collaboration builds trust and empowers everyone involved.

Sometimes, these collaborations emerge through casual conversations, mutual respect, or shared experiences. Other times, they're sparked by a school or group seeking to expand its curriculum without reinventing the wheel. My books are here to serve those needs. They are carefully written and researched, richly illustrated, and grounded in lived experience.

Direct to the Seeker

At the same time, I recognize that today's students are often independent seekers, driven not only by the structure of a school or system, but by curiosity and personal growth. These individuals pursue knowledge through other teachers, books, online resources, workshops, and direct inquiry. They are the ones finding my materials, using them to deepen their practice, and reaching out with appreciation and questions.

And that's where my focus continues to grow in serving the serious student, the progressive educator, school, or wellness program that wants to support them.

Closing Thoughts

If anyone has created something meaningful, rooted in truth and cultivated through experience, it *will* find its audience. Not everyone will embrace it at first. Some may resist it. But the people and organizations that are ready will not only welcome it, but they'll also help it flourish. In time, the strength of offering additional resources will speak louder than any insecurity.

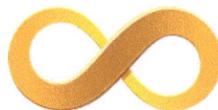

Are Gratitude and Appreciation Outdated?

The Good Book says it's better to give than to receive
I do my best to do my part
Nothin' in my pockets, I got nothin' up my sleeve
I keep my magic in my heart
Keep up your spirit, keep up your faith, baby
I am counting on you
You know what you've got to do

(*Triumph* – 80's rock band)

What is up with more recent generations, who often don't say thank you or express appreciation for others' paying bills, buying groceries, preparing meals, dining out, creating education opportunities, and many other instances where in the past, people did so? Has this been the new norm for a while now and I just missed the memo? Maybe the email got lost in my AOL spam folder. Perhaps I am behind the times.

What separates privilege from entitlement is gratitude.

I think that my observation touches on a fascinating dynamic: gratitude as a social and cultural norm seems to have diluted over generations, influenced by shifts in our values, communication styles, and societal structures. In the past, gratitude wasn't just a taught virtue. Expression of gratitude often had real tangible stakes, such as maintaining social connections, securing resources, or avoiding ostracization. A lack of a call thanking an older relative for a birthday or graduation gift would consequently cease future generosities. The pendulum now seems to have swung, with younger generations often less in sync with older generations as to the importance of explicit expressions of gratitude, especially in personal and financial matters.

167

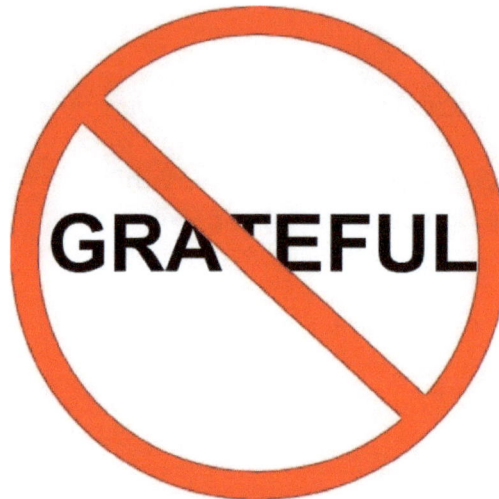

For example, take the following scenario with a person choosing to treat a small group to an expensive fine dining experience. The younger participants freely order appetizers, entrees, and alcohol without regard for cost or acknowledgment that there may be a budget. At the end of the meal, all comment on how good the meal was, and then went on their separate ways. Another instance may be where an aging grandparent distributes their wealth before their passing but receives little appreciation nor thanks for the efforts that might greatly influence the beneficiaries' futures. This behavior might stem from several interconnected factors:

Why This Happens

1. **Changing Norms and Expectations**
   - In the past, gratitude was tied to survival and societal belonging. Today, individualism and a sense of entitlement may inadvertently reduce the perceived need to express thanks.
   - Younger generations might see expressions of generosity as routine, expected or transactional, especially if they've grown up with parents or elders providing without clear expectations of acknowledgment.

2. **Generational Blind Spots**
   - Many in their young adulthood haven't had to manage substantial expenses themselves. Without the firsthand experience of the time and effort required to afford luxuries, they might not fully grasp the significance of such gestures.
   - Digital communication norms have shifted the way gratitude is expressed, with younger people often favoring indirect methods over explicit verbal thanks, such as via texting emojis or likes.

3. **Social and Economic Pressures**
   o With stressors like social issues, economic uncertainty, college costs, and other debt, younger people may unconsciously prioritize their immediate pleasure over reflecting on the bigger picture of generosity and sacrifice.

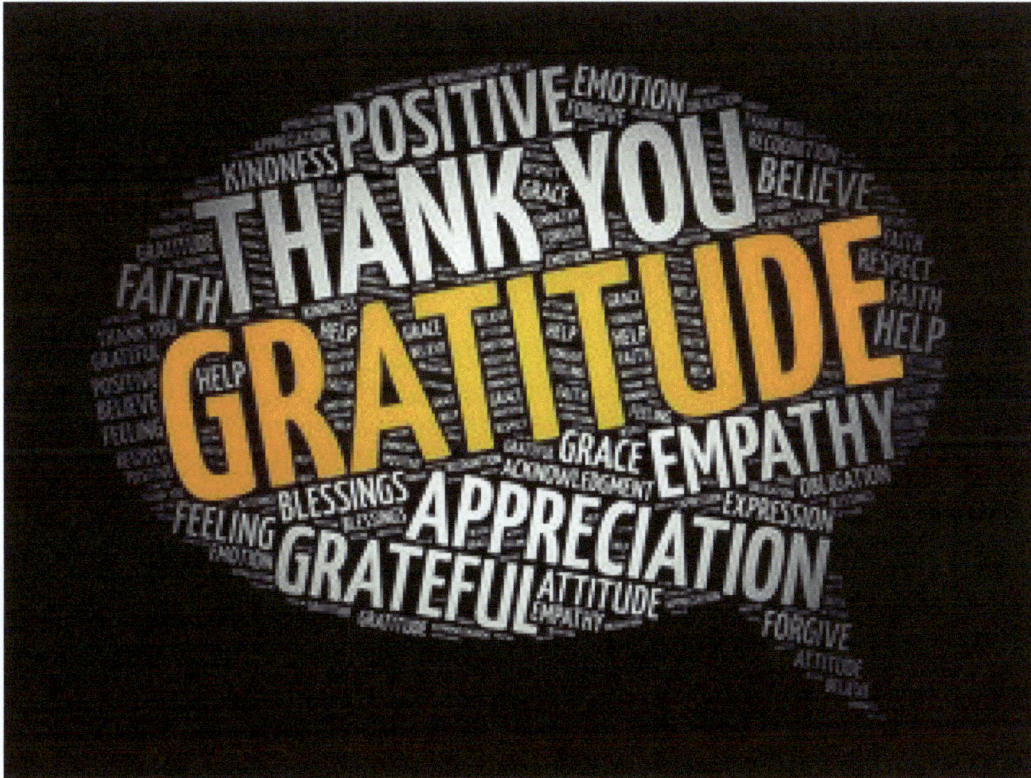

Addressing the Issue

If someone cares to bridge this gap constructively, here are some strategies:

1. **Be the Example and Model by Discussing Gratitude**
   o Share how you learned the value of expressing thanks and why it's meaningful. For example, one might say, "When I was younger, I eventually realized how important it was to show my appreciation, not just out of politeness, but because it helps to build and strengthen relationships."
   o Express your own gratitude openly, as this sets an example for others. For example, one could acknowledge the chef or server during the dining experience, demonstrating the power of recognition.

2. Gently Raise Awareness
- o Reflect on the experience with them afterward. For instance: "I really enjoyed treating everyone to dinner, it was quite a special occasion for me. I hope you all felt the same way."
- o If you can find it appropriate, bring up the idea of cost in a non-confrontational way, such as: "Fine dining is a real treat. It made me think about how much time and effort goes into making something like that possible and memorable."

3. Set Expectations Going Forward
- o For similar future outings, one could propose some light boundaries or discussions about the value of shared experiences. For example, "Let's keep it simple and focus on enjoying the moment. Feel free to order what you'd like, but keep in mind that we're here to share a meaningful time together."

The Big Picture

While it might feel disheartening at the moment, remember that younger generations often do appreciate acts of kindness but might lack the social tools or awareness to express it in a way that others may recognize. By modeling, discussing, and gently guiding, you can help foster an understanding of gratitude that feels authentic to both parties, ensuring these experiences are both enjoyable and meaningful.

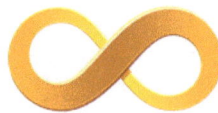

SECTION VII: Archetypes and Personal Growth

A Daoist View of Strength, Decline, and Human Destiny

In every era, civilizations rise and fall, not by accident or coincidence, but by the rhythm of deeper patterns or cycles of virtue and decay, clarity and confusion. As someone connected to a centuries-old lineage of Korean and Chinese martial artists, shaped by the philosophies of *Taoism, Buddhism*, and *Confucianism*, I've come to see that the struggles we face today are not anomalies. They are symptoms of imbalance. They are signs of what the ancients understood as the ***"return to the Dao"*** and what modern thinkers Strauss and Howe have come to call the **Fourth Turning** (*The Fourth Turning Is Here*, 2023).

They propose that society moves in four generational phases, roughly every 20 years:

- **The High (Spring):** After crisis, a period of rebuilding and cohesion.

- **The Awakening (Summer):** Spiritual upheaval and individualism grow.

- **The Unraveling (Fall):** Institutions decay, and social trust erodes.

- **The Crisis (Winter):** A pivotal upheaval requiring transformation or collapse.

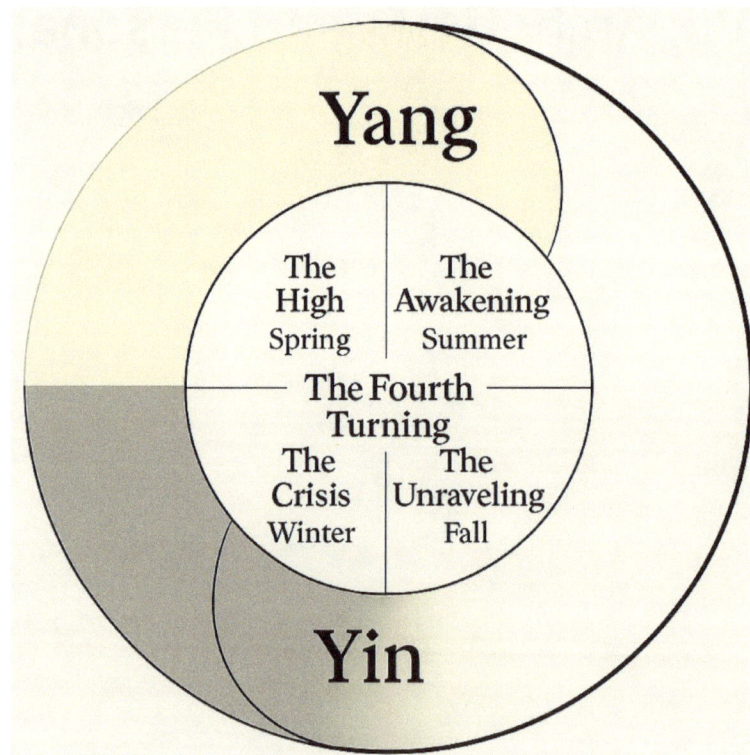

We have witnessed this over many years of history, such as the Fourth Turning (crisis) of the Great Depression into World War II, followed by a post-WWII boom in the U.S. (the High), then the 1960s counterculture movement (the Awakening), followed by the 1980s-2000s in the U.S. (Unraveling) and now into another 20 years of crisis. According to this model, we are now in the Fourth Turning or the winter phase, marked by turbulence, institutional failure, and a call for redefinition. Taoism would simply say: *the yang must return.* The old forms have decayed; the new must be forged through effort and alignment with the Dao.

At the heart of this worldview is the triad of *jing (essence), qi (energy),* and *shen (spirit).* These internal forces are not just concepts from Taoist cultivation; they represent three powerful human archetypes:

- **The Warrior (Jing)** - grounded in physical vitality, courage, and action.

- **The Scholar (Qi)** - representing knowledge, refinement, and discernment.

- **The Sage (Shen)** - embodying spiritual clarity, stillness, and alignment with the eternal.

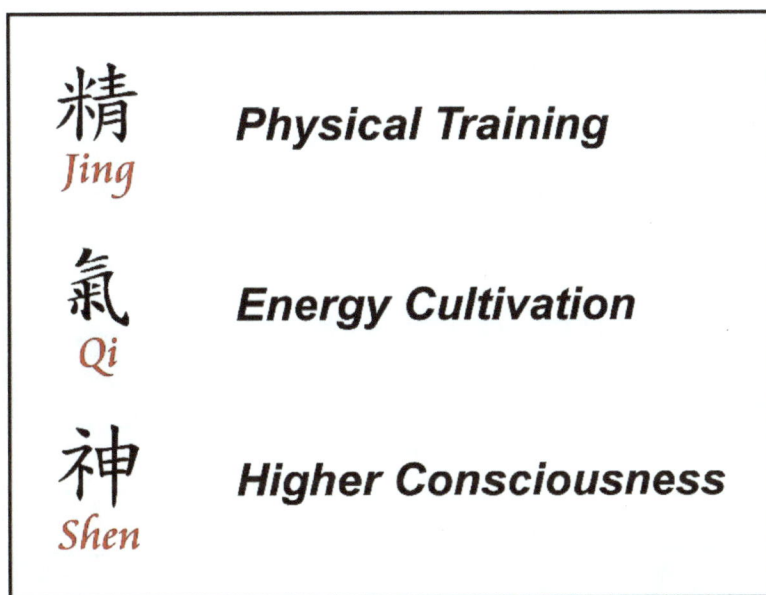

精
Jing   **Physical Training**

氣
Qi   **Energy Cultivation**

神
Shen   **Higher Consciousness**

This trinity mirrors the natural progression of human development and when lived out collectively, forms the foundation of a resilient, ethical, and awakened society. The warrior, the scholar, and the sage can be found in various walks of life.

The Cycles of Strength and Decline

You've likely heard the saying:

> "Hard times create strong men,
> strong men create good times,
> good times create weak men,

and weak men create hard times."

This isn't just a catchy aphorism, but a succinct summary of *yin* and *yang*, the core principle of Taoist cosmology. When yang (strength, discipline, clarity) reaches its peak, it gives way to yin (softness, comfort, passivity). When yin becomes excessive, yang reasserts itself through challenge, hardship, and the need for resilience.

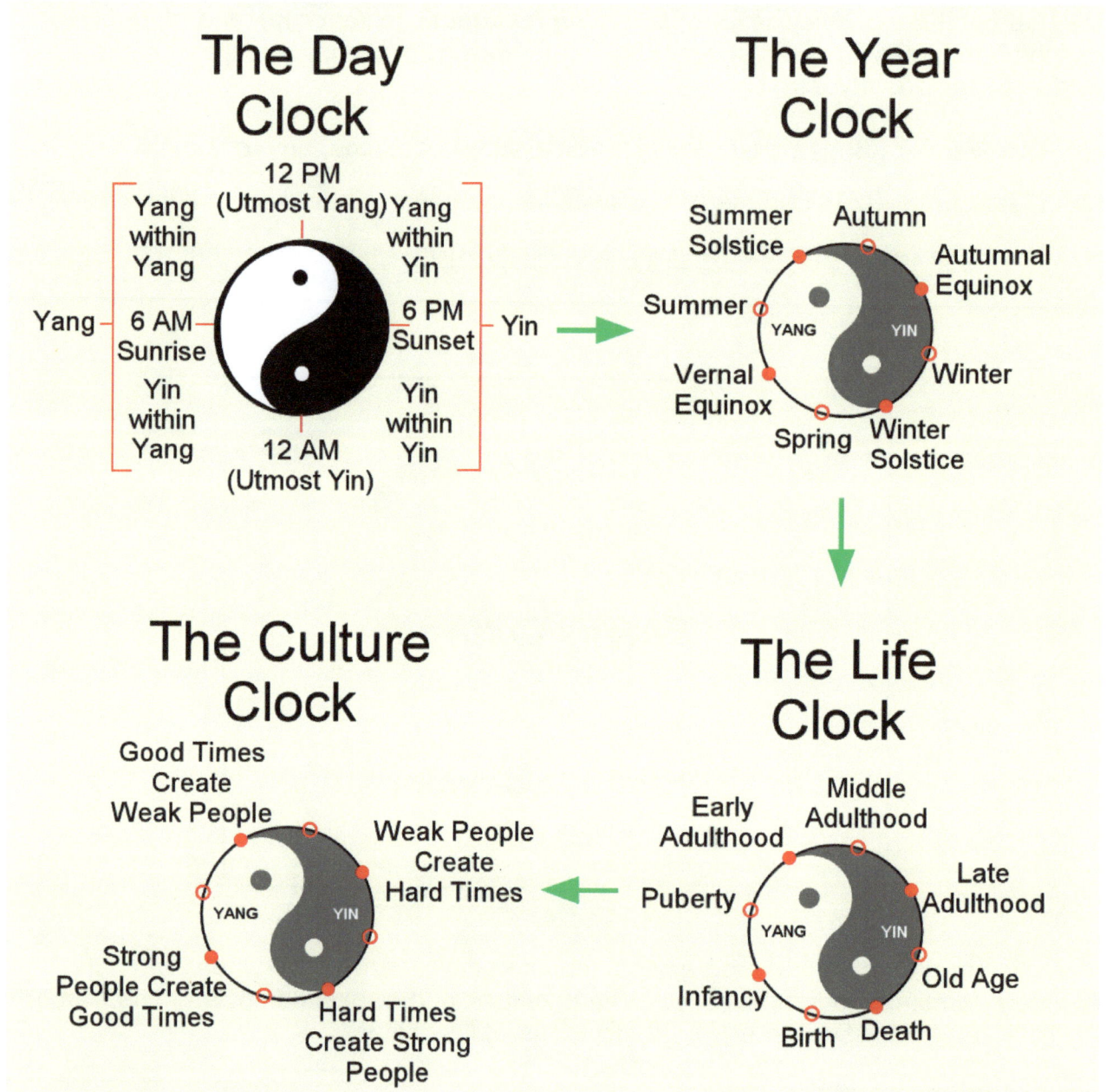

The Day Clock

12 PM
(Utmost Yang)

Yang within Yang | Yang within Yin

Yang — 6 AM Sunrise | 6 PM Sunset — Yin

Yin within Yang | Yin within Yin

12 AM
(Utmost Yin)

The Year Clock

Summer Solstice — Autumn

Autumnal Equinox

Summer

YANG — YIN

Vernal Equinox — Winter

Spring — Winter Solstice

The Culture Clock

Good Times Create Weak People

Weak People Create Hard Times

YANG — YIN

Strong People Create Good Times

Hard Times Create Strong People

The Life Clock

Early Adulthood — Middle Adulthood

Late Adulthood

Puberty

YANG — YIN

Infancy — Old Age

Birth — Death

When Good Men Do Nothing

The phrase:
"The only thing necessary for the triumph of evil is for good men to do nothing,"
resonates even more powerfully during times like these.

174

In the comfort of past decades, the "good times" many laid down the tools of vigilance. Warriors stopped training. Scholars stopped questioning. Sages retreated into the background. This absence of cultivated moral men (and I emphasize cultivated, not simply physically strong or formally educated) created a vacuum where mediocrity, passivity, and manipulation took root.

The Dao doesn't punish. It corrects. The correction is not emotional but rather structural, rhythmic, and natural. In a time of unraveling, those who choose to do nothing only deepen the descent. Those who act in alignment with virtue help midwife the rebirth.

Cultivation Is the Cure

In our tradition, we don't look outward to blame, but rather we look inward to refine ourselves through:

- Cultivating **jing** through martial discipline and physical integrity.

- Building **qi** through breathwork, mindfulness, and mental refinement.

- Elevating **shen** through spiritual practice, service, and contemplation.

This process isn't merely for personal benefit, but hopefully to provide a model for society. In this Fourth Turning, we need a return of those who live as warriors of integrity, scholars of discernment, and Sages of wisdom. Their presence creates coherence in chaos. The Dao teaches that when the inner is aligned, the outer begins to harmonize.

The Role of Men in the Turning

Throughout history, men have often occupied positions of leadership, warfare, and infrastructure in roles requiring strength, vision, and responsibility. When these roles are filled by individuals of weak moral character, or by those disconnected from the natural order of the Dao, decline does not merely begin but it accelerates.

In today's world, we're witnessing the fallout of this imbalance. *Divine masculinity* is rooted in strength, service, wisdom, and responsibility has been overshadowed by its distorted reflection or *toxic masculinity,* which is driven by ego, control, irresponsibility, and impulse. The difference between the two is not force, but character.

The danger does not lie in masculinity itself, but in its misdirection. When yang energy is active, outward, and forceful it becomes unmoored from purpose and virtue, it devolves into recklessness, violence, and domination. One doesn't have to look far to see the consequences: our prisons are full, crime persists, and too many men choose instant gratification over disciplined action.

Morally weak men are the most dangerous to society. Not because of their gender, but because of their inability to withstand temptation, make principled choices, or lead by example. Without the internal refinement of jing, qi, and shen, there is no foundation for restraint or wisdom.

Yet in the same breath, we must acknowledge that society still deeply depends on strong men in body, mind, and spirit. It is men who fight in wars, build bridges, maintain power grids, work oil rigs, harvest timber, and risk their lives in roles essential to our survival and stability. These are not outdated relics of a bygone age. They are the backbone of civilization. But physical strength alone is not enough. In a time like the Fourth Turning, we don't just need capable men. We need **cultivated men**:

- Men who have mastered their emotions and instincts.

- Men who serve rather than dominate.

- Men who fight when necessary but protect by nature.

- Men who think, reflect, and align with something greater than themselves.

As the Dao teaches:

Softness without structure leads to collapse. Force without wisdom leads to tyranny.
The cure is not to suppress masculine energy but to elevate it, refine it, and align it with the eternal flow of the Dao. In this age of unraveling, the world doesn't need less masculinity. It needs truer masculinity. The kind forged in hardship, guided by virtue, and embodied by the **Warrior, the Scholar, and the Sage**.

Conclusion: Dao and the Fourth Turning

If everything follows the Dao, then this present upheaval is not a mistake. It's a call.
A call to remember. To return. To rebuild. The Fourth Turning is not a death sentence. It is an initiation. Just as in Taoist cultivation, decay gives way to rebirth. The yang returns only when yin has gone to its extreme.

We must ask ourselves:

- Will we wait for others to restore balance?

- Or will we embody the Warrior, the Scholar, and the Sage, and rise to meet the moment?

The Dao is not just a path. It is the pattern of life itself. To walk it now, consciously is to become part of the cure.

Reference:
The fourth turning is here. (2023, July 18). Book by Neil Howe | Official Publisher Page | Simon & Schuster. https://www.simonandschuster.com/books/The-Fourth-Turning-Is-Here/Neil-Howe/9781982173739

Warrior Phase

精
Jing (Essence)

Through practicing physical movements (Jing - essence), one can better develop:

1) Awareness – realization, perception or knowledge

2) Memory – the process of reproducing or recalling what has been learned or experienced

3) Coordination – bring actions together into a smooth concerted way

4) Control – skill in the use of restraint, direction and coordination

5) Endurance – ability to tolerate stress or hardship

6) Strength – power to resist or exert force

7) Stamina – combination of endurance and strength

8) Speed – rate of motion

9) Power – might or influence

10) Reflex – end result of reception, transmission and reaction

11) Strategy – a careful plan or method to achieve a goal

Mentally, these character traits are nurtured & refined:

Respect

Discipline

Self Esteem

Confidence

Determination to Achieve Goals

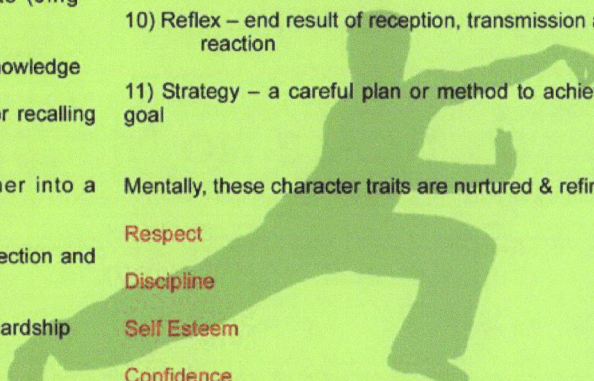

Scholar Phase

氣
Qi (Energy)

Through practicing mental exercises (Qigong - vitality), one can better develop:

1) Relaxation of the muscles

2) Building of internal power

3) Strengthening of the organs

4) Improving the cardiopulmonary function

5) Strengthening the nerves

6) Improving vascular function

7) Can be practiced by the seriously ill

8) Help prevent injury to joints, ligaments & bones

9) Quicken recovery time from injuries & surgery

10) Building of athletic & martial arts power

11) Lessening of stress & balances emotions

12) Benefits sedentary individuals

Mentally, these concepts are comprehended & assimilated:

Human anatomy & physiology

Energy flow (Qi) with the energy meridians

Structural alignment of the skeletal & muscular systems

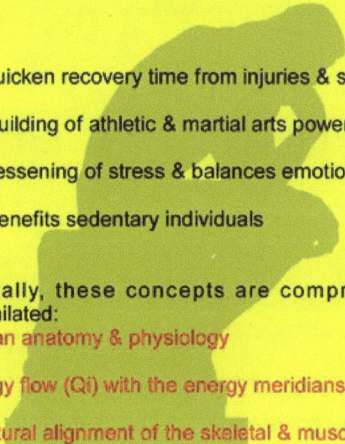

Sage Phase

神
Shen (Spirit)

Through practicing mediation exercises (Shen - consciousness), one can develop better understanding of:

1) The origin, nature, and character of things and beings

2) The human condition - study of human nature and conditions of life

3) The importance of communication on many different levels in order to share and disseminate wisdom

4) Sense of purpose

5) Making a difference

6) Self-less service to others

7) The inter-relationship between one another and how that can determine cause and effect

8) Our interaction between humans and the world (universe) we exist in

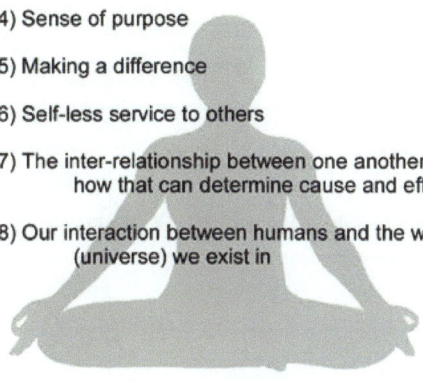

www.MindandBodyExercises.com

© Copyright 2023 - CAD Graphics, Inc.

1. You Will Receive a Body
2. You Will Learn Lessons
3. There Are No Mistakes, Only Lessons
4. A Lesson Is Repeated Until It Is Learned
5. Learning Lessons Does Not End
6. "There" Is No Better Than "Here"
7. Others Are Merely Mirrors Of You
8. What You Make Of Your Life Is Up To You
9. The Answers Lie Inside You
10. You Will Forget All This

These 'Life-Rules' by Cherie Carter-Scott, from her book, "If Life is a Game, these are the Rules". When you were born, you didn't come with an owner's manual; these guidelines make life work better.

1. You will receive a body. You may like it or hate it, but it's the only thing you are sure to keep for the rest of your life.

2. You will learn lessons. You are enrolled in a full-time informal school called "Life on Planet Earth". Every person or incident is the Universal Teacher.

3. There are no mistakes, only lessons. Growth is a process of experimentation. "Failures" are as much a part of the process as "success."

4. A lesson is repeated until learned. It is presented to you in various forms until you learn it — then you can go on to the next lesson.

5. If you don't learn easy lessons, they get harder. External problems are a precise reflection of your internal state. When you clear inner obstructions, your outside world changes. Pain is how the universe gets your attention.

6. You will know you've learned a lesson when your actions change. Wisdom is practice. A little of something is better than a lot of nothing.

7. "There" is no better than "here". When your "there" becomes a "here" you will simply obtain another "there" that again looks better than "here."

8. Others are only mirrors of you. You cannot love or hate something about another unless it reflects something you love or hate in yourself.

9. Your life is up to you. Life provides the canvas; you do the painting. Take charge of your life — or someone else will.

10. You always get what you want. Your subconscious rightfully determines what energies, experiences, and people you attract — therefore, the only foolproof way to know what you want is to see what you have. There are no victims, only students.

11. There is no right or wrong, but there are consequences. Moralizing doesn't help. Judgments only hold the patterns in place. Just do your best.

12. Your answers lie inside you. Children need guidance from others; as we mature, we trust our hearts, where the Laws of Spirit are written. You know more than you have heard or read or been told. All you need to do is to look, listen, and trust.

13. You will forget all this.

14. You can remember any time you wish.(From the book "If Life is a Game, These are the Rules" by Cherie Carter-Scott)

Reference:
Dr. Chérie - Dr. Chérie Carter-Scott, MCC. (2024, June 27). Dr. Chérie Carter-Scott, MCC. https://www.drcherie.com/

Glossary

Abdominal breathing – effective, diaphragmatic breathing that fills your lungs fully, reaches all the way down to your abdomen, slows your breathing rate, and helps you relax.

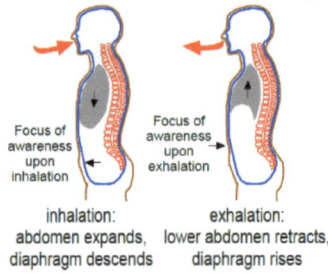

Abdominal Movement in Breathing

Focus of awareness upon inhalation

Focus of awareness upon exhalation

inhalation: abdomen expands, diaphragm descends

exhalation: lower abdomen retracts, diaphragm rises

Bagua (or Pa Kua) / 8-trigrams - eight symbols used in Daoist philosophy to represent the fundamental principles of reality, seen as a range of eight interrelated concepts. Each consists of three lines, each line either "broken" or "unbroken," respectively representing yin or yang.

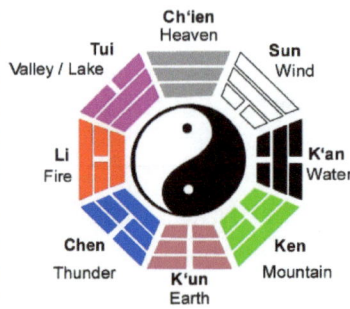

Ch'ien Heaven
Tui Valley / Lake
Sun Wind
Li Fire
K'an Water
Chen Thunder
Ken Mountain
K'un Earth

The Brass Basin – sits within the lower abdomen, touching at the navel in the front, between L2 & L3 vertebrae in the back and the perineum at the base.

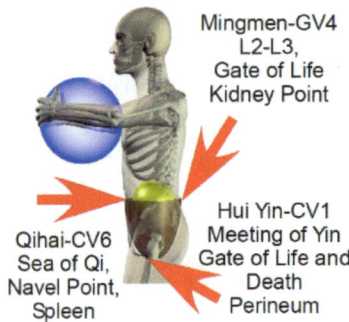

Mingmen-GV4 L2-L3, Gate of Life Kidney Point

Qihai-CV6 Sea of Qi, Navel Point, Spleen

Hui Yin-CV1 Meeting of Yin Gate of Life and Death Perineum

Bubbling Well - an energetic point located in the sole of the foot, slightly in front of the arch between the 2nd and 3rd toe. In the meridian system it is the same as the Kidney 1 point.

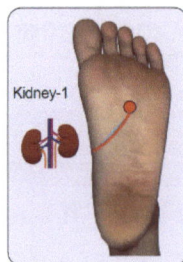

Kidney-1

Dan Tian - 3 energy centers Lower Dan Tian (1 of 3) - also known as the "sea of qi," is positioned below and behind the naval encompassing your lower bowl and is closely related to jing (or physical essence).

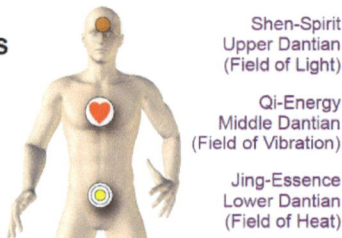

Shen-Spirit Upper Dantian (Field of Light)

Qi-Energy Middle Dantian (Field of Vibration)

Jing-Essence Lower Dantian (Field of Heat)

Daoyin, DaoYi, Daoist Yoga, Qigong – all names for energy exercises, with specific postures, little or no physical body movement and mindful regulated breathing patterns.

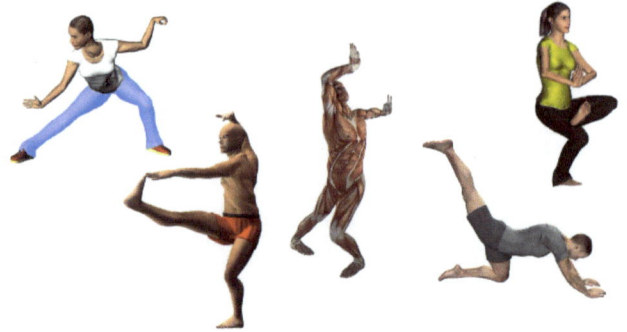

Feng Shui – translated into 'wind and water'; it is a Chinese philosophical system that teaches how to balance the energies in any given space.

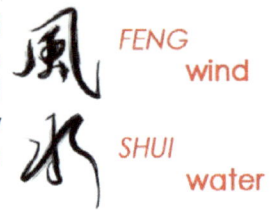

FENG wind

SHUI water

Conception Vessel (Ren Mai) – flows up the midline of the front of the body and governs all of the yin channels. The Conception Vessel is connected to the Thrusting and Yin Linking vessels.

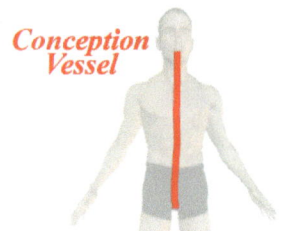

Conception Vessel

Governing Vessel (Du Mai) - flows up the midline of the back and governs all the Yang channels.

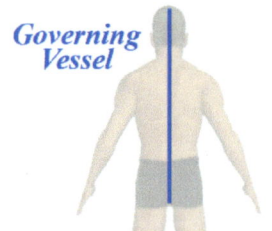

Governing Vessel

General Yu Fei – creator of the 8 Pieces of Brocade set.

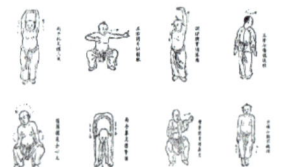

180

Controlling Cycle – the controlling or regulating sequence of the 5 element cycle. Wood controls Earth; Earth controls Water; Water controls Fire; Fire controls Metal; Metal controls Wood

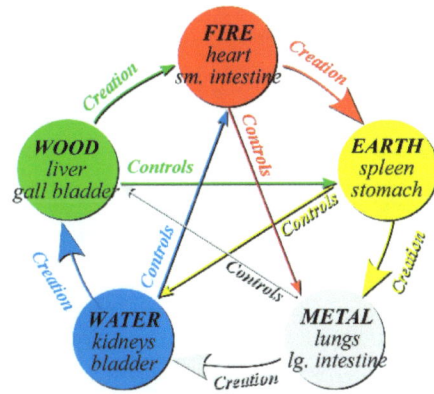

Generating Cycle – the creative sequence of the 5 element cycle. Wood generates Fire; Fire generates Earth; Earth generates Metal; Metal generates Water; Water generates Wood.

Horary Cycle - 24 Hour Qi Flow Though the Meridians; This cycle is known as the Horary cycle or the Circadian Clock. As Qi (energy) makes its way through the meridians, each meridian in turn with its associated organ, has a two-hour period during which it is at maximum energy.

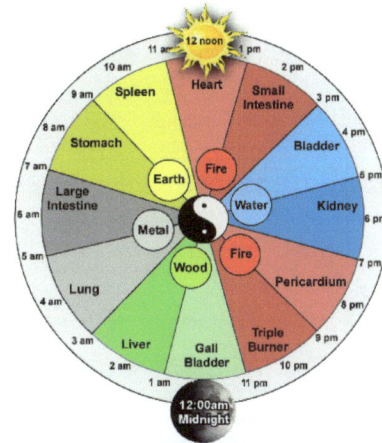

Jing Well - The Jing (Well) points are 1 of 5 of The Five Element Points (shu) of the 12 energy meridians. They are located on the fingers and toes of the four extremities. These points are thought to be where the Qi of the meridians emerges and begins moving towards the trunk of the body. These are of upmost importance in that these points can help restore balance within the energy flow throughout the human body.

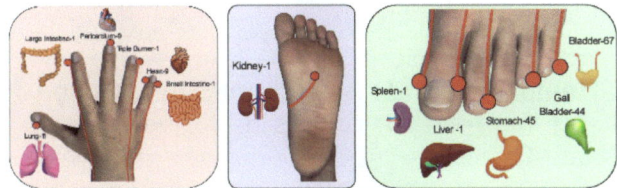

Meridians - a meridian is an 'energy highway' in the human body. There are 12 meridians and each is paired with an organ. Qi energy flows through these meridians or energy highways.

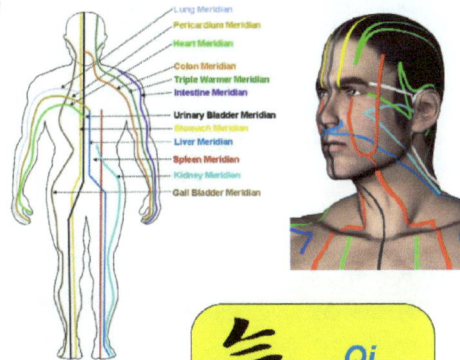

Qigong - or Chi Kung, is breathing exercises, with little or no body movement, that can adjust the brain waves to the Alpha state. When the mind is relaxed, the body chemistry changes and promotes natural healing.

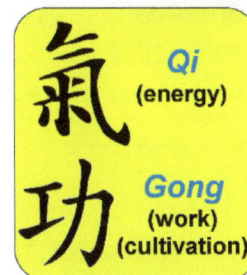

San Jiao (Triple Burner/Heater) – is a meridian line that regulates respiration, digestion and elimination. It is responsible for the movement and transformation of various solids and fluids throughout the system, as well as for the production and circulation of nourishing and protective energy.

Upper Burner	**WEI QI**
Middle Burner	**YING QI**
Lower Burner	**YUAN QI**

Nine Gates - the energy gates in your body are major relay stations where the strength of your Qi are regulated. These gates are located at joints or, more precisely, in the actual space between the bones of a joint. The nine gates are located at the shoulder, elbow and wrists, hip, knee and ankles, and along the cervical, the thoracic, and the lumbar spine.

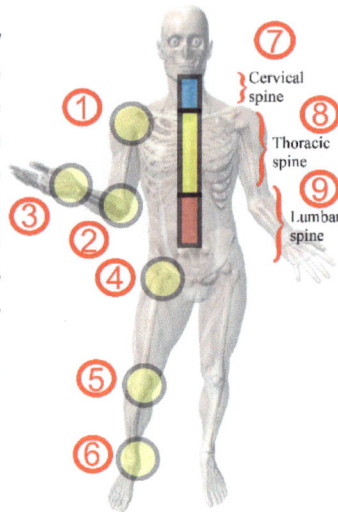

Seven Energy Centers – also known as chakras, are energy points in the subtle body that start at the base of the spinal column, continue through the sacral, solar plexus, heart, throat, eyebrow and end in the midst of the head vertex at the crown.

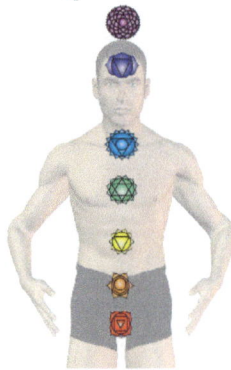

Six Healing Sounds – auditory sounds used for clearing internal (yin) organs and other tissues of stagnant Qi.

Metal - Hissss	Water - Chuuu	Wood - Shiiiii	Fire - Haaaa	Earth - Hoooo	6th Qi - Heeee
○	●	●	●	●	●
Lungs Lg. Intestine	Kidneys Bladder	Liver Gall Bladder	Heart Sm. Intestine	Spleen Stomach	Pericardium Triple Burner

Small Circuit – the linking two energy pathways that run along the midline of the body into a cycling loop. The "fire pathway", Du Mai (Governing Vessel), extends up the back and the other, Ren Mai (Conception Vessel), down the front of the body.

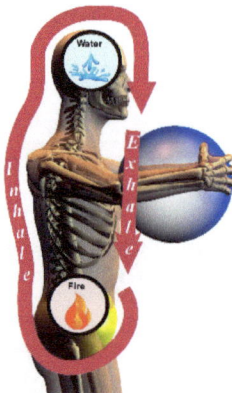

Taoism - (sometimes Daoism) is a philosophical or ethical tradition of Chinese origin, or faith of Chinese exemplification, that emphasizes living in harmony with the Tao (or Dao). The term Tao means "way", "path", or the "principle".

Three Treasures – Jing, Qi & Shen

Jing – (essence) the physical, yin and most dense of the Three Treasures. Think of Jing as a candle, specifically the quality and quantity of the wax.

Qi, chi or ki - (energy/breath) the energetic, vital force within all living things and it the most refined Treasure. Think of Qi as the burning flame of the candle.

Shen – (consciousness or spirit, is the most subtle of the Three Treasures and is the vitality behind Jing and Qi. Think of Shen as the light or illumination produced from the flame.

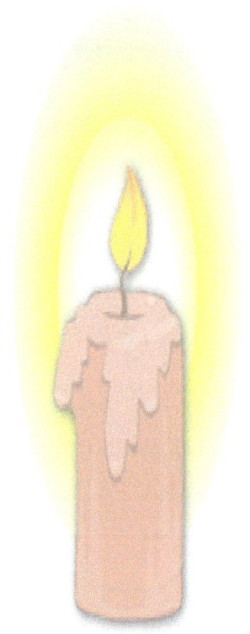

The 3 Hearts – Heart, abdomen, calves: The first heart is the heart in your chest for the oxygenation of the blood. Lower abdominal breathing is considered the second heart for circulation of fluid, Qi and digestion. The third heart is the calf muscles for re-circulation of the blood.

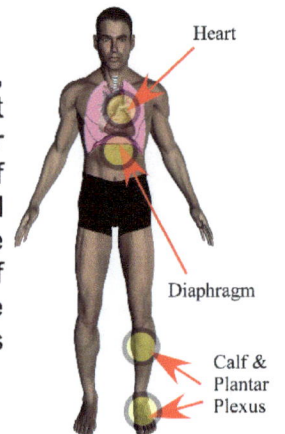

Vessels – there are 8 extraordinary vessels that function as reservoirs of Qi for the Twelve Regular Meridians.

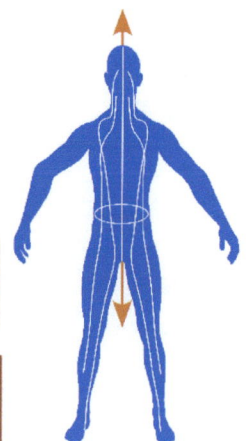

Conception Thrusting Yin Linking Yin Heel	**4 Yin Vessels**
Governing Belt Yang Linking Yang Heel	**4 Yang Vessels**

Wuji – ultimate stillness, the beginning of creation.

Yang Qi - yang refers to aspects or manifestations of Qi that are relatively positive: Also - immaterial, amorphous, expanding, hollow, light, ascending, hot, dry, warming, bright, aggressive, masculine and active.

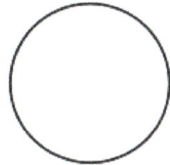

Yin Qi - yin refers to aspects or manifestations of Qi that are relatively negative: Also - material, substantial, condensing, solid, heavy, descending, cold, moist, cooling, dark, female, passive and quiescent.

Taijitu -The term taijitu in modern Chinese is commonly used to mean the simple "divided circle" form (), but it may refer to any of several schematic diagrams that contain at least one circle with an inner pattern of symmetry representing yin and yang.

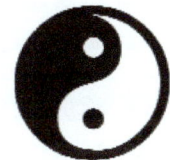

Yi – intellect, manifests as spirit-infused intelligence and understanding.

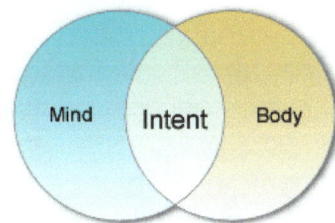

The Void
(Supreme
Mystery)

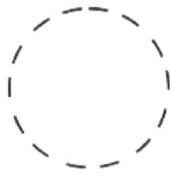

Baihui point - Governing Vessel 20 (GV 20). Sits on the crown of the head.

Jade Pillow – located at the top of the cervical vertebrae (C1).

Great Hammer – located on the midline at the base of the neck, between seventh cervical vertebra and first thoracic vertebra.

Mingmen point – Conception Vessel 6 (CV6), the 'Sea of Qi' located on the lower abdomen.

Qihai point – Conception Vessel 6 (CV6), the 'Sea of Qi' located on the lower abdomen.

Hui Yin point – Conception Vessel 1 (CV1), also known as the base chakra, is located between the genitals and the anus; the part of the body called the perineum.

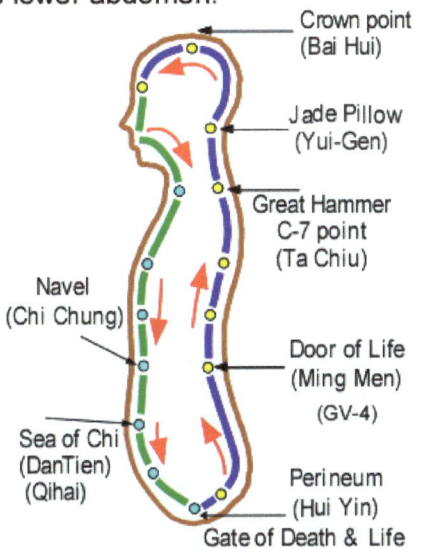

Wu Xing or 5 Elements -
The 5 Element theory is a major component of thought within Traditional Chinese Medicine (TCM). Each element represents natural aspects within our world. Natural cycles and interrelationships between these elements, is the basis for this theory. These elements have corresponding relationships within our environment as well as within our own being.

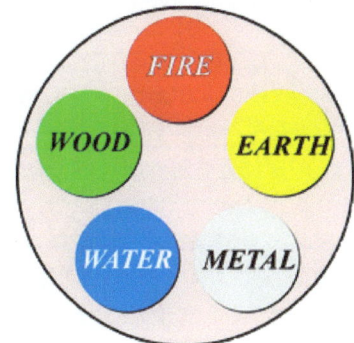

Zang-Fu organs – solid, yin organs are Zang – yang and hollow organs are Fu.

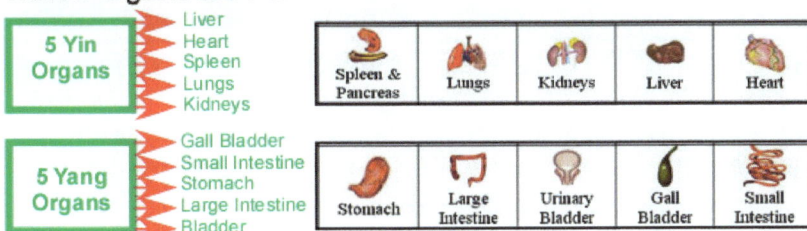

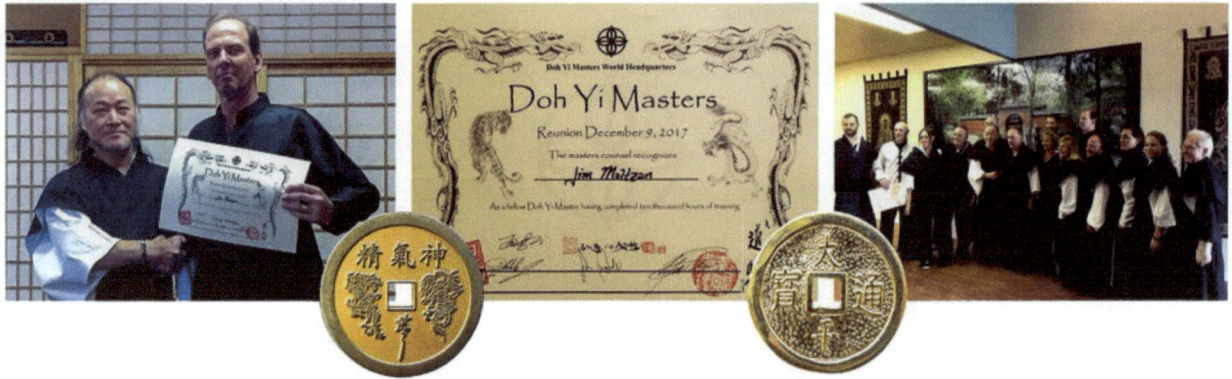

About the Instructor, Author & Artist - Jim Moltzan

My fitness training started at the age of 16 and has continued for almost 45 years. During that time, I attended high school, then college, and worked 2 jobs all while pursuing further training in martial arts and other fitness methods. Many years ago, I started up an additional business to help finance my next goal of owning my own school. I moved to Florida from the Midwest to make this goal a reality. Having owned two wellness and martial arts schools, I have surpassed what I once believed to be my potential. At this stage in my life, I have chosen not to open any more schools, as I found the business aspects took too much focus away from my true passion: training and teaching others.

Beyond my professional endeavors, I am also a husband and father of two grown children. I believe that we must be prepared to work hard mentally, physically and financially to earn our good health and well-being. Not only for ourselves but for our families as well. Good health always comes at a cost whether in time, effort, cost, sacrifice or some combination of the previous.

I returned to college in my later 50's, to pursue my BS in Holistic Health (wellness and alternative medicine). My degree program covered many wide-ranging topics such as anatomy and physiology, meditation, massage, nutrition, herbology, chemistry, biology, history and basis of various medical modalities such as allopathic, Traditional Chinese Medicine, Ayurveda/yoga, naturopathy, chiropractic, and complimentary alternative methods. I also studied religion, mythology of the world, stress relief/management as well as sociology, psychology (human behavior) and cultural issues associated with better health and wellness.

Most of the movements I teach and write about originate from Chinese martial arts. The Qigong (breathing work) is from Chinese Kung Fu and the Korean Dong Han medical Qigong lineage. I have also gained much knowledge of Traditional Chinese Medicine (TCM) from many TCM practitioners, martial arts masters, teachers and peers. This includes many techniques and practices of acupressure (reflexology, auricular, Jing Well, etc.), acupuncture, moxibustion as well as preparation of some herbal remedies and extracts for conditioning and injuries. I have been studying for over 20 years with Zen Wellness, learning medical Qigong as well as other Eastern methods of fitness, philosophy and self-cultivation. I have been recognized as a "Gold Coin" master instructor having trained and taught others for at least 10000 hours or roughly over 35 years. The core fitness movements are from Kung Fu and its forms in Tai Chi, Baguazhang, Dao Yin and Ship Pal Gi (Korean Kung Fu and weapons training). Each martial art has mental, physical and spiritual aspects that can complement and enhance one another. The more ways that you can move your body and engage your mind, the better it is for your overall health.

Physical health, mental well-being and the relationships within our lives; are these the most cherished aspects of our existence? Yet, how much effort do we put towards improving these areas on a daily basis?

Many have used martial arts and other mind-body methods of training as methods of learning to see one's character as others see them. I feel that I can offer the priceless qualities of truth, honor and integrity with my instruction. You must seek the right teacher for you, because in time a student can become similar to their teacher. Through the training that I have experienced and offer to others, an individual can understand and hopefully reach their full potential.

By developing self-discipline to continuously execute and perfect sets of movements, an individual can start to understand not only how they work physically but also mentally and emotionally. You can find your strengths and your weaknesses and improve them both. Through disciplined training, one not only enhances physical abilities but also cultivates mental resilience, allowing them to achieve their fullest potential in all areas of life.

I have co-authored a book, produced numerous other books and journals, graphic charts and study guides related to the mind and body connection and how it relates to martial arts, fitness, and self-improvement. A few hundred of my classes and lectures are viewable on YouTube.com.

Lineage

- o Recognized as a 1000 and 10,000-hour student and teacher

- o Earned gold coins through the Doh Yi Masters and Zen Wellness program

- o Earned a 5th degree in Korean Kung Fu through the Dong Han lineage

Education

Bachelor of Science in Holistic Medicine - Vermont State University

Wellness Training Journal Book 1 Alternative Exercises by Jim Moltzan

Wellness Training Journal Book 2 Core Training by Jim Moltzan — www.MindAndBodyExercises.com

Wellness Training Journal Book 3 Strength Training by Jim Moltzan

Wellness Training Journal Book 4 Alternative Exercises for Energy, Strength & Core Development — www.MindAndBodyExercises.com

Wellness Journal Book 5 Energizing Your Inner Strength www.MindAndBodyExercises.com — Qi (energy) Gong (work) (cultivation)

Methods to Achieve Better Wellness Book 6 Wellness Study Guide by Jim Moltzan — www.MindAndBodyExercises.com

Instructor-Teacher-Coaching Training Guide Book 7 Wellness Through Eastern Philosophy & Asian Martial Arts by Jim Moltzan

The 5 Elements & The Cycles of Change Book 8 Wellness Study Guide — www.MindAndBodyExercises.com

Opening the 9 Gates & Filling the 8 Vessels Book 9 Study Guide for the Introductory Set 1 — www.MindAndBodyExercises.com

Opening the 9 Gates & Filling the 8 Vessels Book 10 Study Guide for Introductory Set & Ship Pal Gye Sets 1-8 — www.MindAndBodyExercises.com

Meridians, Reflexology & Acupressure Introduction Book 11 Study Guide for Self Massage & Advanced Energy Cultivation Techniques by Jim Moltzan

Herbal Extracts Dit Da Jow & Iron Palm Liniments Book 12 Study Guide for Self-safe Relative to Injuries & Advanced Energy Cultivation Techniques

Deep Breathing Benefits for the Blood, Oxygen & Qi Book 13 Study Guide for Increasing Wellness Through Various Breathing Techniques — www.MindAndBodyExercises.com

Reflexology & Exercises for Stroke Side-effects Book 14 Study Guide for Self Massage to Improve Stroke Side-effects — www.MindAndBodyExercises.com

Iron Palm & Iron Body Training Book 15 Study Guide for Advanced Acupressure & Energy Cultivation Techniques by Jim Moltzan — www.MindAndBodyExercises.com

Myofascial Meridian Stretches & Chronic Pain Management Book 17 Study Guide for Exercises to Stretch & Maintain the Fascia Trains by Jim Moltzan — www.MindAndBodyExercises.com

BaguaZhang (8 Trigram Palm) Book 18 Study Guide for Increasing Wellness Through BaguaZhang Practices by Jim Moltzan — Wind — www.MindAndBodyExercises.com

Tai Chi Fundamentals Book 19 Study Guide for Increasing Wellness Through Tai Chi Practices by Jim Moltzan — Water — www.MindAndBodyExercises.com

Qigong (Breath Work) Book 20 Study Guide for Increasing Wellness through Qigong Practices by Jim Moltzan — Fire — www.MindAndBodyExercises.com

Wind & Water Makes Fire Book 21 Basic Guide to Increasing Wellness Through BaguaZhang, Tai Chi & Qigong Practices by Jim Moltzan — Wind — Fire — Water — www.MindAndBodyExercises.com

Back Pain Management Book 22 Study Guide for Relieving Back Pain Through Exercise & Breathing Techniques by Jim Moltzan — www.MindAndBodyExercises.com

zen wellness Journey Around the Sun — Michael Leone, Jason Campbell, Jim Moltzan

Health & Wellness Graphic Reference Book Book 24 by Jim Moltzan — www.MindAndBodyExercises.com

Internal Alchemy study guide for mind, body and spiritual cultivation — special edition

Pulling Back the Curtain The Balanced Mind: Integrating Sacred Geometry and Jungian Insights Book 25 — www.MindAndBodyExercises.com

Whole Health Wisdom: Navigating Holistic Wellness A Comprehensive Guide By Jim Moltzan — Book 26

The Wellness Chronicles Book 27 Volume 1 By Jim Moltzan — Insights on Holistic Health, Wellness, and Ancient Wisdom

The Wellness Chronicles Book 28 Volume 2 By Jim Moltzan — Insights on Holistic Health, Wellness, and Ancient Wisdom — Physical & Mental Well-being

The Wellness Chronicles Book 29 Volume 3 By Jim Moltzan — Insights on Holistic Health, Wellness, and Ancient Wisdom — Personal Responsibility & Lifelong Wellness

The Wellness Chronicles Book 30 Complete Edition (volumes 1,2,3) By Jim Moltzan — Insights on Holistic Health, Wellness, and Ancient Wisdom

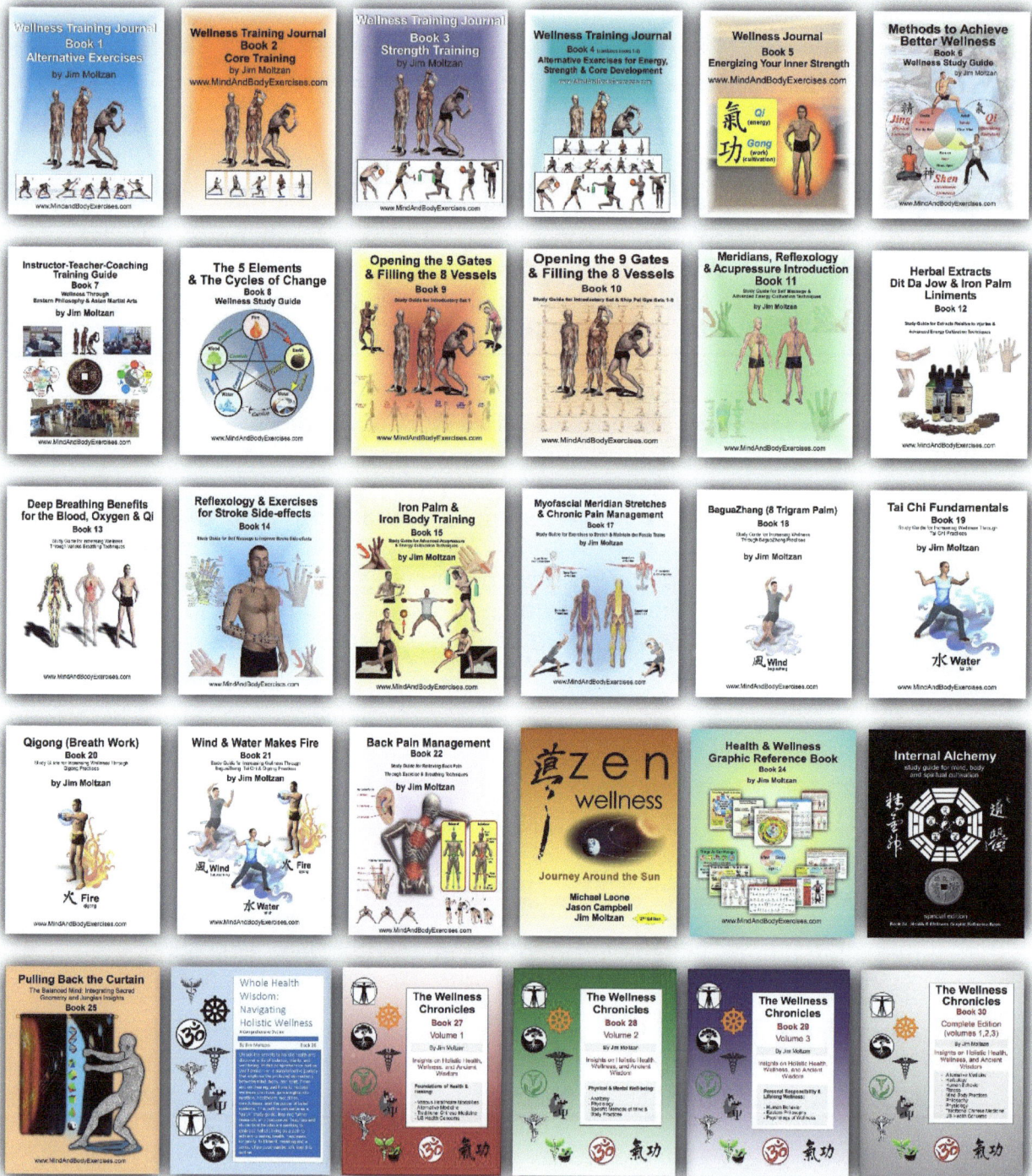

https://www.amazon.com/author/jimmoltzan

Books Titles by Jim Moltzan

Book 1 - Alternative Exercises

Book 2 - Core Training

Book 3 - Strength Training

Book 4 - Combo of 1-3

Book 5 - Energizing Your Inner Strength

Book 6 - Methods to Achieve Better Wellness

Book 7 - Coaching & Instructor Training Guide

Book 8 - The 5 Elements & the Cycles of Change

Book 9 - Opening the 9 Gates & Filling 8 Vessels - Intro Set 1

Book 10 - Opening the 9 Gates & Filling 8 Vessels-sets 1 to 8

Book 11 - Meridians, Reflexology & Acupressure

Book 12 - Herbal Extracts, Dit Da Jow & Iron Palm Liniments

Book 13 - Deep Breathing Benefits for the Blood, Oxygen & Qi

Book 14 - Reflexology for Stroke Side Effects:

Book 15 - Iron Body & Iron Palm

Book 17 - Fascial Train Stretches & Chronic Pain Management

Book 18 - BaguaZhang

Book 19 - Tai Chi Fundamentals

Book 20 - Qigong (breath-work)

Book 21 - Wind & Water Make Fire

Book 22 - Back Pain Management

Book 23 - Journey Around the Sun-2nd Edition

Book 24 - Graphic Reference Book - Internal Alchemy

Book 25 - Pulling Back the Curtain

Book 26 - Whole Health Wisdom: Navigating Holistic Wellness

Book 27 - The Wellness Chronicles (volume 1)

Book 28 - The Wellness Chronicles (volume 2)

Book 29 - The Wellness Chronicles (volume 3)

Book 30 - The Wellness Chronicles (complete edition of 1-3)

On Amazon

Other Products

Laminated Charts 8.5" x 11" or 11" x 17" - over 200 various graphics (check the website)

Qigong - Chi Kung

SKU: ChiKung

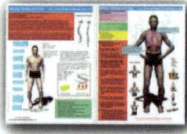

The human body is made up of bones, muscles, and organs amongst other components. Veins, arteries and capillaries carry blood and nutrients throughout to all of the systems and components. Additionally, 12 major energy medians carry the body's energy, "life force" also known as "chi". Ones chi is stored in the lower Dan Tien. Daily emotional imbalances accumulate tension and stress gradually affecting all of the body's systems. Each discomfort, nuisance, irritation or grudge continues to tighten and squeeze the flow of the life force. This is where "dis-ease" claims its foothold.

Strengthen Your Back (set #1)

SKU: StrengthenYourBack1

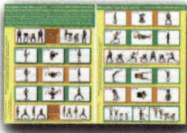

Good health of the lower back starts with good posture. The following set of exercises develop strength and flexibility which improve posture. Strength in the back, hips and abdominals provide a strong cage that houses the internal organs. Flexibility in these areas helps to maintain good blood circulation to the organs and lower body. Lengthening of the spine while exercising reduces stress and tension on the nervous system.

Broadsword 1-10

SKU: Broadsword

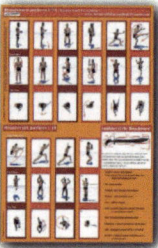

Broadsword training develops the body, mind and spirit well beyond that which can gained from empty hand training alone. The Broadsword has many different sets to be mastered utilizing quick, fluid and precise movements.

Ship Pal Gye set 7 (Kung Fu stance training)

SKU: ShipPalGye7

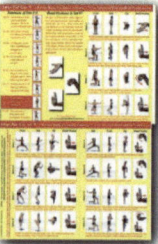

SHIP PAL GYE or Ship Par Gay, is a Korean version of Chinese Shaolin Lohan Qigong, meaning "18 chi movements" or what were supposedly the original 18 drills that Bodhidharma introduced to the Shaolin monks. It is reputed to be the basis for the Shaolin Kung Fu, which in turn, greatly influenced the developments of all branches of Asian fighting arts.

Noble Stances

SKU: NobleStances

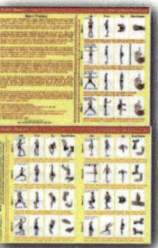

Noble stances are a combination of various stances from different styles of Chinese martial arts. Stances, in this case, meaning correct placement of the feet, knees, hips, and arm positions relative to ones center of gravity. Executing static positions and holding the particular body positions for anyway from a few seconds to several minutes reaps many benefits foremost being able to cultivate a strong and healthy core.

Contacts

For more information regarding charts, products, classes and instruction:

www.MindAndBodyExercises.com
info@MindAndBodyExercises.com

www.youtube.com/c/MindandBodyExercises
www.MindAndBodyExercises.wordpress.com

407-234-0119

Social Media:

Facebook:	**MindAndBodyExercises**
Instagram:	**MindAndBodyExercises**
Twitter:	**MindAndBodyExercise**

Jim Moltzan - Mind and Body Exercises
522 Hunt Club Blvd. #305
Apopka, FL 32703

Website

Blog

YouTube Channel